Nature's Gym

Conquer Every Season and Every Weather

by

Oliver Hamilton

Table of Contents

Introduction: Embracing the Outdoors 1

Chapter 1: The Allure of Nature's Gym 4

Chapter 2: Spring into Action 12

Chapter 3: Summer's Fiery Energy 23

Chapter 4: Autumn's Transition... 33

Chapter 5: Winter's Wonderland 43

Chapter 6: Rain or Shine: Adapting to Wet Weather 53

Chapter 7: Wind's Dynamic Resistance... 61

Chapter 8: Snow and Ice: Extreme Elements.................................... 68

Chapter 9: Finding the Right Equipment... 78

Chapter 10: Personalising Your Nature's Gym Routine 85

Chapter 11: Staying Motivated Through the Seasons........................ 92

Chapter 12: Nutrition for the Seasons 102

Chapter 13: The Solitary Explorer 109

Chapter 14: Group Dynamics: Social Sweat Sessions 117

Chapter 15: Families Outdoors: Inclusive Fitness 124

Chapter 16: City Meets Nature: Urban Outdoor Fitness.................. 131

Chapter 17: Wild and Free: Exploring Remote Landscapes 138

Chapter 18: Nighttime in Nature's Gym.............................. 145

Chapter 19: Mindfulness and Wellness in the Great Outdoors........ 152

Chapter 20: Thrill-Seekers and Adrenaline Junkies.................. 159

Chapter 21: Healing through Nature................................. 166

Chapter 22: The Nature's Gym Success Stories 173

Chapter 23: The Environmental Footprint of Fitness 180

Chapter 24: Weathering the Storm:
When Outdoor Isn't an Option 188

Chapter 25: The Future of Outdoor Fitness......................... 196

Chapter 26: The Year-Round Call of the Wild 203

Appendix A: Seasonal Checklists and Planning Tools................ 207

Appendix B: Resources for Further Reading and Exploration......... 210

Appendix C: Safety Guidelines and First Aid Tips 213

Appendix D: Weather-Appropriate
Recipes for Outdoor Athletes...................................... 216

Introduction:
Embracing the Outdoors

There's something inherently rejuvenating about stepping outside, filling your lungs with fresh air, and setting your sights on the horizon. It's as if the world is extending an open invitation to explore, to move, and to connect with the environment in a way that feels fundamentally human. This book—your guide to finding vigor and vitality through the great outdoors—charts a course for this very adventure.

Imagine the outdoors as a boundless gym, without walls and with a sky for a roof. Each element plays a part in your well-being. The earth underfoot steadies you, the breeze challenges you, and the sun energises you. It's the kind of gym that is inclusive and ever changing, where the activities morph with the seasons and the scenery provides an ever-refreshing backdrop to your fitness journey.

From the quiet hush of a snow-blanketed landscape to the energetic buzz of a sunny, green park, nature invites us into its myriad gym spaces. Whether it's the serene challenge of a mountain hike or the playful skirmish of a beach volleyball match, this book is about seizing those opportunities to enliven both body and mind, no matter the season. It's about feeling empowered to step out the door, come rain, shine, or the in-between.

Yet engaging with the outdoors isn't just about physical exercise; it's a multi-faceted experience. It's the silent communion with the dawn chorus on a misty morning run, the ripples of laughter with friends on a summer's day trek, and the swish of leaves during an autumnal cycle. The outdoors nurtures us, teaches us, and offers a canvas on which we can chart our personal growth.

The call of the wild is an all-year affair. Spring's tender light nudges you to set intentions and renew your goals, mirroring the fresh blossoms and vibrant new growth around you. Summer's zest lends itself to peak activity, urging you to soak up the sun's fiery energy. Autumn's kaleidoscope of colours is a visually arresting reminder to adapt and embrace change, and winter, with its crisp air, whispers tales of resilience and introspection. There's no off-season in nature's gym—only phases, each with its own allure and lessons.

As we weave through the chapters of this guide, we won't merely discuss the mechanics of outdoor exercise or offer prescriptive regimes. Instead, we will delve into the sensory, emotional, and sometimes transcendental moments that occur when we engage physically with the natural world. We shall discover how each element and every weather condition has something to offer, whether it's the resistance of the wind or the refreshing slap of rain against the skin.

Nature doesn't hoard its treasures; it lavishly displays them for those willing to participate. From urban parklands to secluded mountain trails, the great outdoors is an open-access sanctuary for everyone. Whether you're a city dweller hungry for a taste of the wild or a rural inhabitant with nature at your doorstep, this book aims to guide you to find balance and rejuvenation amidst the elements.

Embracing the outdoors is not just for the seasoned athlete or the adventure enthusiast. It's for every one of us. It's for the early risers, the night owls, the solitude seekers, and the social butterflies. This book will encourage you to find a routine that resonates with your soul, one that infuses wellbeing into each day, and transforms challenges into opportunities. Your outdoor journey is deeply personal, and this guide is here to support that quest.

Motivation can ebb and flow like the tide, it's natural. Yet, even when the fervour wanes, the outdoors remains a steadfast ally. It does not judge but consistently offers fresh starts and merciful reprieves. We'll explore how to harness this perpetual source of inspiration, turning nature into both a coach and a confidant, pushing you towards your best self.

Through tales of transformation and testimonies of triumph, you'll see that the fabric of outdoor fitness is woven from stories as diverse as the landscape itself. The book will share various narratives that illuminate how the fusion of fitness and nature can be a catalyst for profound personal change.

Throughout these pages, there's also a quiet acknowledgment of responsibility. As you draw strength and solace from the outdoors, there lies an implicit duty to safeguard it. We'll touch upon sustainable practices and the importance of treading lightly, ensuring that our footprints on this earth are gentle. The environment that serves as your gym also serves as home to countless others; respecting it is paramount.

The harmony between the human spirit and the rhythm of nature is ancient, yet it awaits rediscovery by each of us. This book is an invitation to step onto that path. So lace up your boots, gear up for all weathers, and let's set forth on this transformative journey. May you be inspired to embrace the outdoors with every fibre of your being, for it promises to embrace you back, in ways you've yet to imagine.

Welcome to your first step outside. Welcome to the journey of a lifetime. It's time to embrace the outdoors with open arms and an open heart. Are you ready?

Chapter 1:
The Allure of Nature's Gym

Step outside and you've entered the most ancient of gyms, where the treadmill is the mountain trail and weights are found in logs and stones. In this welcoming environment, you don't just exercise your body; you engage with the world, your senses invigorated by the rustle of leaves and the crunch of gravel underfoot. There's something profoundly alluring about nature's gym—it's an open invitation to challenge your physical limits while finding harmony with the natural world. Here in the open air, fitness isn't confined to repetitive motions within mirrored walls. It's dynamic, adapting to the roll of the landscape and the whisper of the wind, an orchestra conducted by the elements themselves. So lace up your boots, gear up, and let's embark on a journey to discover how nature's varied terrain can sculpt our bodies, sharpen our minds, and attune us to the earth's rhythm.

The Mind-Body-Nature Connection

Turning our gaze to the synergistic relationship between mind, body, and the natural world, we uncover a tapestry of connections woven through our every sensory experience. The great outdoors isn't merely a backdrop for physical exertion; it is a dynamic, interactive space that engages and enhances our mental faculties as it does our muscles. Our emotional states, cognitive abilities, and physiological responses are intrinsically linked with the natural environments we immerse ourselves in. This isn't hocus-pocus; it's the hard-won wisdom of feet trampling trails, of breaths drawn deep amidst forests and mountaintops.

Envision the body as an orchestra, each organ and limb a section that plays in perfect time. But the maestro of this symphony – to bring forth true harmony – must be the mind. It sets the tempo for our engagement with the elements, nudges us to leap through the stinging cold rivers, and pushes us to hike the extra mile. And as we do, our heartbeat crescendos, our muscles rise in fortissimo. But notice the subtler tunes too: the calming serenades of serenity and the curious vibratos that nature stimulates.

Science lends support to what adventurers have long known: spending time in nature isn't a mere luxury; it's a critical component of our health and wellbeing. It's the act of syncing one's own rhythm with the pulse of the natural world. When we step outside, our senses flare to life – the fragrant smells, the rustle of leaves, and the uneven texture of the ground beneath our feet. This feast for the senses helps reduce stress hormones, lighten the burden of anxiety, and lift our mood.

As we lace up our trainers and step out of the door, our bodies begin the anticipatory dance of adrenaline and endorphins. But the story doesn't end with chemicals and cardiovascular gains. Movement in natural spaces requires a more nuanced navigation, a deeper engagement of the mind in balance and spatial awareness. This cognitive challenge not only sharpens our reflexes but also strengthens our mind-body connection, cementing a more grounded presence within ourselves.

Take the patterns of the seasons, for example, they are not just calendars to us but guides to weave variety into our fitness regimes. The rolling of seasons enthral us, be it the fresh sprouts of spring that beckon us to renewal, the blazing heat of summer asking for our endurance, the falling leaves of autumn teaching us to let go, or the white stillness of winter calling for our quiet strength. Each comes with its own mental engagement, each is a new chapter in the unfolding story of our personal wellbeing.

It's paramount to recognise the physiological benefits that echo long after a workout concludes. When our exercise is entwined with nature, recovery periods evolve into more than muscle repair. They become moments for our neural pathways to embed the day's physicality, fusing the sensory inputs with motor output, tightening the weave of our personal tapestry of movement and thought.

Then there's the dimension of meditation in motion. The Zen found in the steady cadence of a jog through wooded trails, or in the rhythmic cycle of paddling across a mirrored lake. In these moments, the chatter of an overloaded mind fades away, replaced by a euphoric tranquillity that sharpens focus and deepens the meditative quality of our exercise.

However, the mind-body-nature connection extends beyond the bounds of self-improvement, spiraling outward to our relationships with others and to the environment. When we move in natural spaces, we forge a non-verbal dialogue with the flora and fauna, the very terrain. This connection tends to foster a sense of stewardship and respect for the earth we tread upon and the air we breathe.

It's this very connection that also drives us to understand the impact of our footprint — not just in the figurative sense, but also the ecological one. Embracing nature as our gym becomes not just a pursuit of health but a sustainable practice, a harmony of vitality and preservation.

Inevitably, life sometimes nudges us indoors, whether due to inclement weather or personal circumstances. Yet, the imprint of nature's influence on our mind and body does not easily fade. Indoor training can still draw on the mental strategies honed outside, the resilience formed in wild winds and the adaptability fostered by unpredictable terrains.

As we consider the journey ahead through the changing landscapes and seasons of our lives, the mind-body-nature connection stands as a pillar of continuity. It's a wellspring of inspiration to adapt our workouts, to align our goals with the ever-shifting colors and contours of the great outdoors.

Connecting with nature isn't simply a method of fitness; it's a holistic approach to life. It's an all-season, all-weather philosophy that harnesses the essence of the natural world to sculpt our physique and refine our psyche. It's as much about nurturing a rich inner life as it is about achieving a vigorous outer form.

And so, the mind-body-nature connection remains an open invitation — a call to step into the expanse, to welcome the elements as one would greet a trusted coach. It's a chance to learn the art of balance, fortitude, and grace amidst nature's own rhythms. It holds the prospect of discovering the purest form of joy: that of being completely present and alive within our bodies as they move through the realm of the living world.

In the pages to follow, we'll further distil the essence of our relationship with the elements, crafting a comprehensive strategy for fitness throughout the seasons. Yet, as we do, this foundation of the mind-body-nature connection will remain central, informing every step, breath, and heartbeat of our journey in nature's vast and open gymnasium.

Harnessing the Elements for Your Fitness

Moving from the mind-body-nature synergy previously discussed, let's dive into the ways you can use the very elements around you to enhance your fitness routine. Imagine for a moment the earth beneath your feet, the wind against your face, the warmth of the sun on your back, and the fresh air filling your lungs. These aren't just poetic sentiments—they're tools at your disposal, free of charge, ready to be leveraged in pursuit of health and vitality.

Firstly, consider the very ground you stand on—whether it's the uneven terrain of a forest floor or the soft resistance of beach sand. Every step on these natural surfaces engages your muscles differently than flat, man-made floors. It's not just physical; it's cerebral. Your brain works harder to navigate the uneven terrain, improving your coordination and proprioceptive abilities. You're not just running; you're adapting, growing stronger, mentally and bodily.

Many shy away from venturing out on a windy day, but here's a thought: why not use that wind as a natural resistance trainer? Just like a swimmer pushing against the current, you can work against the wind to increase the intensity of your workouts. It's unpredictable, yes, but that unpredictability forces you to engage core muscles for balance and stability, giving you a workout that's both organic and invigorating.

Don't underestimate the power of a good dose of sunshine, either. Moderate exposure to sunlight boosts vitamin D levels, vital for bone health and immune function. Pair that with an outdoor jog or yoga session, and you're transforming your fitness routine into a holistic health ritual.

Cold weather is another factor often seen as a deterrent. However, when properly prepared with the right layers, working out in the cold can be incredibly refreshing. It stimulates your circulation, increases calorie burn, and if you're keen on winter sports, offers a fun and exhilarating form of exercise that doubles as a skill. It's about embracing the crisp air and finding joy in the puff of your breath visible in the morning chill.

Further to the physiological benefits, embracing the elements for your fitness challenges your mental fortitude. It's easy to roll out of bed and onto a yoga mat indoors, but stepping out into the rain for a run demands a toughness that pays dividends in discipline and resilience. Once you've splashed through a few puddles or felt the rain on your skin as you exercise, you realise it's not just a workout; it's an adventure.

Let's not forget the rivers and seas—water workouts can be a serene form of fitness. From swimming to paddleboarding or kayaking, working out on or in water not only sculpts your physique but also offers meditative tranquillity. The resistance of water is gentle on the joints while being remarkably effective for building strength and endurance.

But what about air quality? It's all very well running outside, but the purity of the air you breathe contributes to your overall wellness. Sometimes, this means seeking out green spaces away from urban pollution. Parks, nature reserves, and trails offer a much-needed breath of fresh air—quite literally—for city dwellers looking to detox their lungs as they tone their bodies.

What about those moments when the sky opens up while you're mid-workout? Don't let the rain wash out your fitness plans. Savour the feeling of raindrops cooling your skin as you build muscle and stamina. Whether it's gentle drizzle or a downpour, it's undeniably invigorating and adds a layer of intensity to your regime.

There's a profound beauty in attuning your workout to the cycles of the day. Sunrise and sunset provide not only spectacular backdrops but also opportunities to bask in the quieter moments of the day. The peaceful ambiance at these times can ground your exercise in a deeper sense of connection with the world around you.

As for the gear—you don't need the latest high-tech gadgets to harness the elements. Indeed, the simplicity of stepping outside negates the necessity for sophisticated equipment. A decent pair of trainers, appropriate clothing for the season, and you're all set to turn the great outdoors into your personal gym.

Moreover, the benefits of harnessing the elements for your fitness extend beyond the corporeal. There's a mental clarity that comes from being immersed in the elements, a kind of meditation in motion. Whether it's the rhythmic patter of rain while you cycle or the hush of a snowy landscape as you ski, these experiences are as much about nurturing your psyche as your physique.

Nature's temperamental ways mean that no two workouts will be the same. You'll face different challenges and enjoy a diverse range of experiences that keep your routine exciting and fresh. It's the opposite of the monotony of a gym treadmill, each outdoor workout chapter unfurls with its unique story to tell.

Finally, as you take your fitness journey into the great outdoors, you'll find yourself becoming more in tune with nature's rhythms. This isn't just a fad or a phase; it's a lifestyle change that aligns with a more sustainable, environmentally conscious way of living. Your workout stops being just about you and starts being about a larger connection to the planet.

The elements are a gift to those who choose to embrace them. They are transformative, challenging, and brimming with the potential to enhance your fitness in ways a gym simply cannot mimic. With each gust of wind, every ray of sunlight, and all the diverse terrain underfoot, they beckon you to step outside and be revitalised.

So, when you close this chapter, look out your window. Whatever the weather, it's perfect for something. Tie up your laces, zip up your jacket, and step into a world of dynamic and elemental fitness. It's right there waiting for you; all you need to do is grab the opportunity and run with it—literally.

Chapter 2:
Spring into Action

As the chilled veil of winter thaws to the vital sunbeams of spring, it's time we too shed our layers of inertia and *spring into action*. This vivacious season is all about renewal—a perfect cue for revamping our workout routines and stepping back into nature's rejuvenating embrace. It's a time when the air buzzes with possibility and the earth sprouts with new promise. **Let's sync our intentions with the season's energy of growth**, curating fitness agendas that are as fresh as the proverbial May flower. With paths carpeted in blooms and a palette of green unfurling before our eyes, our natural gymnasium beckons with open arms. The elixir of crisp mornings is not just about aesthetically pleasing landscapes—it's a call to enliven our senses, re-energize our bodies, and nourish our minds. So pull your trainers out, restring your hiking boots, and lay out your yoga mat amidst the daffodils; it's time we burgeon alongside nature, making each stride, pedal, or stretch a personal testament to this season of boundless potential.

Renewal and Growth: Setting Intentions

After exploring the vitality and potential of embracing the outdoors as your gym, we now turn a fresh page towards spring—a symbolic and literal time for renewal. This period, often spilling over with ephemeral blooms and invigorating air, offers us an opportunity to plant seeds for future growth. Setting intentions is not merely about outlining goals, but also about aligning our aspirations with the natural cycle of rebirth and progression that spring exemplifies.

Why set intentions rather than simply goals? Imagine your goal as the distant mountain peak, formidable and distinct. The intention, then, is the compass in your hand—the mindset and values that guide every step towards that peak. As you embark on this phase, consider which aspects of your wellbeing you're most eager to nurture—perhaps endurance, strength, or maybe inner tranquility. Each intention should resonate with your core, creating a personal springtime cadence that'll flow into your outdoor activities.

To foster this growth, we must engage in reflective groundwork. Take a walk among the budding trees, feel the soft, yielding earth, and breathe in the crisp, reviving air. Allow the sensory experience of nature to permeate your thought process, guiding your mind towards clarity. Here, in the midst of nature's awakening, ask yourself what you would like to awaken within you. Is it a long-lost hobby, a skill, or a new fitness milestone?

While the season gently nudges us towards action, remember that setting intentions is as much about patience as it is about ambition. It's about understanding the rhythms of nature and our place within it. Recognising that growth is not instantaneous but progressive; akin to the way a seedling doesn't erupt into a tree overnight, our personal development requires consistent nurturing and time.

Much like the tender shoots that wrestle through the soil to find the sun, our intentions need to be anchored into tangible plans. Begin by sketching out how your fitness activities will interweave with the landscape's transformation. This could be as structured as a bi-weekly hike to observe the changing scenery or as fluid as incorporating an additional outdoor yoga session to soak up the increasing warmth.

Your intentions should also be reflexive, adapting to both your own growth and nature's shift. As the season flourishes, take note of how your body and psyche respond to your outdoor regimen. Are your spirits lifted by the longer daylight hours? Does the chirping choir of dawn inspire you to rise earlier for a run? Let these inherent springtime motivators integrate with your intentions, energising your actions.

Setting intentions also allows for personal discovery and pushing past perceived limits. It is spring, after all, a time of exploration and experimentation. Plan to venture off your usual track, try a new exercise, or engage with a different aspect of the natural world. Perhaps the previously unnoticed path offers a different terrain that could improve your agility or the local river beckons for a bout of kayaking?

During this chapter of renewal, focus on fostering a resilient mindset. Envision your intentions weaving resilience into your daily practices. As spring's unpredictable weather patterns rollout— sunshine one day, showers the next—let your adaptability bloom. You might find that resilience in the outdoors mirrors a broader capacity to handle life's oscillations.

It's essential in this intention-setting process to also foster communal and environmental consciousness. Share your renewed spirit and intentions with others, inviting camaraderie on treks or jogs. This not only builds a supportive network but deepens your connection with others who also find solace and strength in the great outdoors.

Moreover, setting intentions with an awareness of the surrounding life also means taking responsibility for it. As you grow, ensure that your activities safeguard the environment. Whether it's adhering to trails to avoid trampling new growth, or picking up litter along your path, each action done with intention fosters a healthier world for all.

As you transition into practical choices to realise your springtime intentions, consider how you'll reflect these aspirations in your gear selection and commitment. Meticulously planning your all-weather gear for spring activities, as discussed in the following section, will be instrumental to support your growth.

Remember that to experience renewal and growth you must not only set intentions but revisit and revise them. Like the unpredictable spring showers that may alter the path you jog on, be prepared to shift your focus if certain intentions no longer serve you. Adaptability is a form of growth, one that's perfectly at home in this ever-changing season.

Lastly, as you tie your laces for that journey along the dew-sparkled trail, take pride in this step towards your intentions. Each bound forward is a commitment, a small victory in the face of the vastness of your potential. The ultimate renewal is the one that happens within, sparked off by the setting of intentions—intentions that guide you through each sprint, each breath, and each moment under the open sky.

As we wrap up this invitation to set intentions, remember that just as nature bursts forth with life, your endeavours can bloom in a myriad of ways. Wrapped in the refreshing embrace of the season, allow this fresh start to infuse every step of your journey. Let the spring be a tapestry of growth, woven with threads of ambition and sewn together with the resilient fibers of intentions. Take this time to align with nature, and your true path will unfold before you with every sunrise and sunset you greet in Nature's Gym.

Springtime Workouts: Blossoming Fitness

As we turn the page from the brisk winds and chills of winter to the warming embrace of spring, our exercise routines are due for a seasonal shift. It's in this spirit of rejuvenation that we take our fitness regimes outdoors, aligning our sweat sessions with the blooming life around us. The fresh air invites us to breathe deeper, and as the world around us awakens, so too does the opportunity for a flourishing fitness routine.

Spring heralds in longer days, and with it, the chance to infuse early morning or late evening workouts with golden rays. Let's consider the dawn exercise, where the quiet world serves as your personal studio. The sun's gentle rise coaxes you into your stride, whether it's a jog around the dewy park or a dynamic stretch session by a tranquil lake. This time of day is magical, offering crisp air and the soundtrack of nature stirring to life.

The versatility of spring weather also prompts a varied workout. On milder days, a hike through budding trails can build endurance as much as it soothes the soul. When mild showers grace the earth, don't be hasty to duck indoors. Embrace the rain, as it turns your routine into a refreshing adventure. With each droplet that cools your skin, you could be dancing through puddles, adding bursts of playful sprints, and feeling the raw joy of nature's shower.

As flowers poke through the softening soil, let it remind you of growth – your own physical and mental fortitude. It's time to push through personal boundaries, perhaps by adding resistance to your runs with a weighted vest or pioneered paths up hills or through uneven terrain that challenge your balance and strength. Each hillock conquered is akin to growth, parallel to the blooming vistas around you.

Bike rides take on a new charm come spring, as the landscapes transform week by week. It's not only about the cardiovascular benefits but also about witnessing the gradual painting of the canvas that is nature. A cycling session becomes an exploration, a willing venture into the artistry of spring's hand.

Group fitness, too, finds its niche in the great outdoors during spring. Enlisted friends can add a layer of encouragement and camaraderie to exercising. You may find a local boot camp setting up in a nearby park, or perhaps it's time to start your own. Group yoga in the open air brings a communal sense to your practice, as you root yourself amidst the energy of budding life.

Speaking of grounding, don't forget the benefits of barefoot workouts on soft grass or sandy shores. The Earth's natural textures massage and activate different muscles in your feet and legs - muscles that are usually dormant due to the perpetual wearing of shoes. Emerging science praises the advantages of grounding and its potential in reducing inflammation and boosting recovery.

For those of you keen on building muscle, the natural world is replete with opportunities. Park benches become platforms for step-ups or tricep dips, trees are sturdy anchors for resistance bands, and playgrounds serve as makeshift gymnastic rings. It's a blend of creativity and functionality, using what's at hand to sculpt and strengthen.

While focusing on physical prowess, let us not neglect the subtle art of balance and flexibility. Spring's unpredictable terrain - from slick, rain-soothed paths to soft, uneven fields - becomes your studio. Practice your yoga, pilates, or tai chi here, as you align your body's movements with the breath of fresh air and allow the uneven ground to deepen your concentration and enhance your stability.

One can't discuss spring fitness without touching on the joy of water sports as they return to favor. Kayaking, paddle boarding, and even open-water swimming wake up with the season, offering both a chilling rush and a full-body workout. The water reflects the sky's changing moods; thus, every venture out is a unique dialogue between you and the elements.

Let's also talk technology, albeit briefly, because it's tempting to count steps, log runs, and quantify every aspect of health. But spring invites you to disconnect. Let the journey through a bed of wildflowers or alongside a murmuring brook be measured in sensations and sights, not just data. Your body will tell you all you need to know, from the warming of your muscles to the zest of energy that post-exercise euphoria brings.

Outdoor fitness enthuses your workouts with an unpredictable element that no gym can replicate. It could be a sudden breeze that challenges your balance in a tree pose, a minor incline that adds to your run's resistance, or the sun peeking from behind the clouds, warming your skin as you catch your breath. Embrace these gifts from nature, and let them grow your adaptability and resilience.

Always attune yourself to the environment's rhythm. Pay attention to the birdsong, the rustle of leaves, the scents carried by the wind. These natural cues sharpen your sensory acuity and can deepen the connection between mind, body, and environment, enhancing the meditative effects of a good workout.

And finally, remember that spring showers not just rain but opportunities - to start afresh, to renew your commitment to health, to explore the outdoors with vigour and view your workouts through a lens of play rather than duty. As branching trees extend into the sky, so should you reach for your fitness goals with a newfound zest for life's natural gym.

With each passing day, nature scripts a narrative of growth and beauty, a backdrop for your blossoming fitness journey. From the first pink flush of dawn to the serene twilight, let every heartbeat of your springtime workouts resonate with the pulse of the living world. After all, isn't that what draws us out here – the undeniable call of the wild that urges us to be healthier, happier, entirely home in the great outdoors?

All-Weather Gear Guide for Spring

- Transition seasons can be a peculiar time for the outdoor enthusiast. The unpredictability of spring weather demands a versatile gear kit that'll help you stay committed to your fitness goals, come rain or shine. Let's dive into the essential components you should consider when sculpting your spring-active wardrobe. Starting with arguably the most important piece, the waterproof jacket – this item isn't just about keeping rain at bay. Opt for a breathable, lightweight version that doesn't turn into a personal sauna as the effort levels rise. A good rule of thumb is to check for underarm vents and adjustable cuffs for that essential air circulation.

- Next, we can't ignore the base layers. They're your second skin, after all. In spring, these need to be adept at moisture management; they should wick away sweat yet provide warmth when the chill lingers in the air. Materials like merino wool or advanced synthetics are perfect, as they can retain heat even when damp while remaining light on the skin. It's also smart to opt for tops with a quarter-zip, allowing temperature regulation as your workout fluctuates between strenuous climbs and mindful meditations.

- Moving downwards, your legs will thank you for investing in quality trousers or leggings that can resist a sudden drizzle. Water-resistant materials are a plus, but avoid anything too heavy. You're looking for gear that can comfortably transition from a sunny jog to a breezy hike without feeling bulky or limiting movement. And let's not forget trousers with zip pockets – secure spots for your keys and phone are non-negotiable during any outdoor pursuit.

- You might not consider gloves and hats as spring essentials, but early mornings and late evenings can still bite. A light pair of gloves and a flexible beanie will suffice for most temperate regions. They're easy to stow away when not needed, but you'll be grateful for them when that unexpected cold front rolls in.

- A good pair of waterproof shoes is crucial - it's the foundation of your outdoor undertakings. They should offer support and have a good grip for those slippery when wet moments. But they should also be breathable; your feet are going to start sweating as much as the rest of you once you get moving. Reflective details aren't amiss either, as the days elongate but darkness can still fall swiftly during early spring evenings.

- Speaking of reflective details, let's talk visibility. If you're out in the dim light of dawn or dusk, high-visibility vests or strips on your clothing are invaluable. Safety doesn't stop at visible gear, though. The transition months bring about changing terrain – icy patches may linger, and wet leaves can be treacherously slippery. Be mindful of where you step and adjust your pace accordingly.

- Accessories come into their own during spring. A running belt or light daypack is essential for carrying the extra gear that the season's capricious nature necessitates. Waterproof casings for electronics, a spare lightweight hat, gloves, or even a compact change of clothes might become necessary mid-adventure.

- Your headwear choices also extend to protection from the sun. A breathable cap can shield you from unexpected heat waves and is easily tucked into a pocket or pack. And don't forget the sunglasses. Spring sun, especially reflected off water or remaining snow, can be intense, and protecting your eyes is as important as protecting your skin – so yes, slap on that sunscreen as well!

- Hydration systems shouldn't be underestimated. Whether you prefer a water bottle or a reservoir in a backpack, make sure it's something that doesn't disrupt your activity, is easy to access, and – ideally – insulated to prevent water from becoming too cold or too warm.

- With unpredictable weather patterns, layering is the name of the game in spring. A lightweight fleece or a pullover can provide the extra insulation needed and can be easily removed and packed away. Go for one that's quick-drying and made of non-absorbent material, because no one enjoys the clamminess of a soaked-through sweater.

- On heavier rainfall days, don't shy away from waterproof trousers or gaiters, especially if trail running or hiking is on the agenda. They might not win any fashion contests, but they're practical for keeping you dry and can be handy to stop ticks or other spring-active critters from finding their way to unwelcome places.

- In terms of materials, while the functionality of synthetics is undebatable, there's a growing trend in seeking sustainably sourced and produced gear. Eco-friendly options are popping up that don't compromise on performance, so keep an eye out for those and contribute positively to the environment you so love to play in.

- And one final note – do your homework on the spring forecast of the area you'll be exploring. Gear might need tweaking if you're moving from a typically mild climate to a mountainous region where winter lingers longer. Pack intelligently, using weather apps and local insights to guide you.

- Remember, the right gear doesn't just keep you comfortable; it bolsters your safety and increases the enjoyment factor of every outdoor endeavor. Spring, with all its freshness and unpredictability, offers a distinctive chance to test your adaptability in Nature's Gym – so embrace it with the right equipment, and you're set for a sublime season of fitness and exploration.

- Staying prepared isn't about expecting the worst; it's about making the most of every moment outside. With these tips folded into your packing list, you're ready to step out into the spring air, confident that whatever the skies serve up, you're equipped to handle it – and thrive.

Chapter 3:
Summer's Fiery Energy

As the earth tilts on its axis, welcoming the unabashed blaze of summertime, we're gifted with the longest days and the shortest nights - it's nature's own invitation to maximise our sunlight hours with heart-pumping, sweat-dripping outdoor workouts. But let's not forget, this is the season that will test your resolve with its searing heat and humidity; remind yourself that it's less about beating the heat and more about embracing and adapting to it, a perfect metaphor for life's challenges. It's the ideal time to swim with the rhythm of the waves, cycle through the warm, heady air, or explore mountain trails that offer up the scent of pine and the song of cicadas as your natural gym soundtrack. As you attune your body to the radiant energy of the sun, remember to find your balance between vigor and virtue – it's about pushing limits, yes, but also ensuring cooldowns and hydration breaks are as much a part of your routine as the crunches and miles. Summer is your moment to glow with vitality, to be fierce yet playful in your pursuits, and to allow the fiery energy of the season to fuel both your body and spirit.

Peak Sunshine: Maximising Outdoor Training

As the embers of the day begin to glow with the promise of summer's warmth, it's time to shift our focus to squeezing every last drop of daylight for our outdoor training. With the sun riding high, we find

23

the golden hours of summer stretching before us, inviting us to step outside into the light and heat.

The key to unlocking summer's full potential is to understand and respect the power of peak sunshine. These long days are a double-edged sword, offering ample time for an array of activities yet presenting the challenge of higher temperatures. To thrive rather than merely survive, it's essential to align our workouts with the sun's arc across the sky.

Morning training sessions can be a revelation, with the air still cool and the world slowly stirring to life. It's a time for peaceful solitude or for sharing the dawn chorus with fellow early birds. As the sun's rays are gentle, this is the perfect window for lengthy runs or bike rides, your body fuelled by the promise of a new day.

And then there's the evening, when the sun dips and the heat begins to ebb away. This is the moment for those who revel in the afterglow of the day, the gym-goers who swap fluorescent lights for the canvas of sunset skies. Whether it's hill sprints or yoga sequences, the descending sun provides a backdrop that fuels the spirit as much as the exercise nourishes the body.

But what of the hours in between? The midday sun may be too potent for maximal exertion, but it's not to be wasted. This is the time for water sports, when the cool relief of the lake or sea beckons. From paddleboarding to swimming, the water provides resistance and refreshment in equal measure.

Hydrate, hydrate, hydrate. Can't stress it enough—the summer's sweltering heat demands a surcharge of fluids. And I'm not just talking about the water you guzzle during your workout. Prehydration is a thing; start sipping before you sweat, keep your water bottle close during your exertions, and don't forget to continue afterwards. Your muscles will thank you, and your recovery will be all the sweeter for it.

Finding refuge in shaded trails or parks can also help you stay cool. The dappled light beneath a canopy of leaves offers a reprieve from the sun's intensity. Positioning your workout in these green pockets allows you to run, leap, and lunge in a cooler setting—a natural retreat from the heat.

Let's not overlook the attire. Clothing plays a pivotal role in staying cool and protected; think lightweight, breathable fabrics, and clever sweat-wicking technologies. And, of course, the quintessential accessories of the savvy summer athlete: sunglasses and a visor or hat to shield your eyes and face from the sun's relentless glare.

Peak sunshine hours also herald unique opportunities for cross-training. It's a season when the water isn't the only element you can use for your regimen. The beach volleyball court, outdoor climbing wall, or even the impromptu boot camp at your local park could be your new favourite gym spot. The rigidity of indoor routines gives way to playful yet powerful workouts.

It's vital, too, to heed the sun's silent alarm. The skin is your largest organ, and protecting it with sunscreen and lightweight long-sleeves is non-negotiable. It's as crucial to your outdoor training regime as the exercises themselves; skin care is self-care, after all.

For those truly looking to capitalise on the extended daylight, the concept of "solar loading" may intrigue. This is the strategic soaking up of sun rays to bolster your vitamin D stores, which play a critical role in muscle function and recovery. But bear in mind, a dab of sun here and there suffices; no need to bake in the blaze for hours on end.

Challenge yourself with a change of pace or terrain. The dry trails of summer offer a stable surface for speed work, letting you push the limits safely. Simultaneously, the pliable sand on the beach offers resistance training for your lower body, crafting strength with each stride against the shifting ground.

The season's heat nudges you towards a fresh consideration of timing and intensity. It's wise to temper summer's eagerness with a touch of prudence—high-intensity interval training (HIIT) can reach new peaks when timed to avoid the midday scourge, and longer, steadier workouts drift towards the cooler bookends of the day.

And don't forget rest. Summer might seem like a sprint, with its flurry of activities and bountiful sunshine, but it's also the season to embrace the art of stillness. Your outdoor training is enhanced by the moments you allow yourself to sit, breathe, and simply absorb the world around you—each rest as important as the movement it punctuates.

Savouring peak sunshine for maximising outdoor training is a balance of enthusiasm and wisdom, a melding of preparation and spontaneity. So lace up your trainers, fill your water bottle, and step into summer's embrace with a plan to sizzle—sensibly.

Staying Hydrated and Safe in the Heat

As we embrace summer's fiery energy, attention must turn to the fundamentals of staying hydrated and safe in the heat. The sun's zenith brings a vibrant intensity to outdoor activities, but it's crucial to navigate the higher temperatures with awareness and care.

Hydration, the elixir of life, becomes especially paramount as the mercury rises. A well-hydrated body functions like a well-oiled machine, but when you're sweating under the sun, keeping your fluid levels topped up is akin to refuelling a race car on the go. Water isn't just a thirst-quencher; it's vital for maintaining blood circulation, muscle function, and temperature regulation.

To prevent dehydration, start hydrating before you feel thirsty. Thirst is a distress signal, indicating that you're already on the path to dehydration. Consider carrying a water bottle during your expeditions and sipping regularly. On longer excursions or intense workouts, titrate your fluid intake with the ambient temperature and your exertion levels. There's a balance to strike, though; overhydration can be just as dangerous as dehydration.

For those days when the heat index skyrockets, timing is everything. Dawn and dusk offer the goldilocks conditions for exertion – not too hot, not too cold, just right. If you can, schedule rigorous activities for earlier in the morning or later in the evening, when the sun's intensity wanes. The air is not only cooler but often carries the freshness of daybreak or the calm of twilight.

Apparel is another potent ally against the oppressive heat. Lightweight, breathable, moisture-wicking fabrics can make a significant difference, allowing your skin to breathe and sweat to evaporate. Some apparel even comes with UV protection, which is worth considering as it can shield your skin from the sun's more harmful rays.

At times, the landscape itself can provide respite. Seek out shaded trails or parks, where trees and buildings offer sanctuary from the relentless sunshine. These oases are not only cooler but enhance the visual pleasure of your workout, framing your exertions against a backdrop of dappled light and leafy vistas.

Remember, too, that your body is your most honest advisor. Heed its signals – if you start to feel lightheaded, dizzy or particularly fatigued, it's a signal to slow down, seek shade, and hydrate. Heat exhaustion and heatstroke are serious risks that can escalate rapidly, so learning to recognise and respond to the telltale signs is of utmost importance.

Electrolyte balance must also be in the equation. When we sweat, we don't just lose water but salts as well. Sodium, potassium, magnesium - these all play a critical role in cell function and hydration.

There are various ways to replenish them: from electrolyte-infused drinks to more natural alternatives like ripe bananas or a pinch of salt in your water bottle.

If a dip in the pool or a sprint through the sprinklers isn't an option, consider carrying a spray bottle filled with water for a quick cool-down. A fine mist over your face and neck can have an astonishingly refreshing effect, immediately lowering your body temperature and providing instant relief.

As for nutrition, favouring lighter meals that include fruits and vegetables with high water content can contribute to your hydration. Melons, cucumbers, strawberries, and peaches do more than tantalise your taste buds; they also give you an extra H_2O boost.

Remember hydration extends beyond pure water. Herbal teas and other non-caffeinated beverages can hydrate without the diuretic effects of caffeine. These can be especially refreshing when served cold and can be a pleasing alternative for those who find water monotonous.

Finally, the buddy system is invaluable. When possible, partake in outdoor activities with a friend or a group. Not only does this tend to make the experience more enjoyable, but it also means an extra pair of eyes to monitor for signs of heat-related issues. There's a comforting safety in numbers, and you can remind each other to take hydration breaks.

Certainly, summer's warmth is no cause for trepidation; it's an invitation to revel in the power of the sun – a reminder of life at its most vibrant. With these strategies to stay hydrated and safe, you're well-equipped to thrive in the heat, to celebrate the season's exuberance while respecting the power of the sun.

These measures aren't just practical checkpoints; they're the practices that sketch out the fine line between endurance and enjoyment. Embracing summer's heat with vigilance allows you to continue venturing into nature's gym, fostering a deeper, safer connection with the great outdoors.

Maintaining well-being through the sizzle of summer, then, is less about battling the elements and more about dancing with them. Understanding the symphony of your body's needs, and the rhythm of nature's heatwave, means you can move to the beat of the bright season, fully engaged and blissfully aware of the sensual delights it offers.

Creating a Balanced Summer Exercise Regimen

As we wade deeper into the warm embrace of summer, it's crucial to tailor our exercise routines to sync with the season's fiery energy. When the mercury climbs, a smart exercise strategy that respects the sun's intensity while taking advantage of the longer days is key—think less about beating personal records and more about embracing the essence of summer.

The cornerstone of any balanced regimen is variety. Just as a well-rounded diet provides multiple nutrients for optimal health, a mixed bag of exercises ensures all muscle groups get attention, reducing the risk for injury from repetitive strain. Incorporate strength training, cardio, flexibility, and restorative activities into your week. The summer season offers ripe opportunities to adapt these elements in alignment with Mother Nature's tempo.

Let's begin with strength training. Seek out calisthenics parks or use playgrounds early in the morning to avoid the heat; outdoor bodyweight exercises can be incredibly effective. Consider doing exercises like pull-ups on branches or dips and push-ups on park benches. If you have access to a beach, the soft sand provides extra resistance, intensifying workouts like squats and lunges—just ensure your form stays on point to avoid undue strain.

For cardio, the extended daylight hours offer a golden chance for early morning jogs or post-work cycling. Always be armed with water to stay hydrated, and favour routes with some shade. And why not throw in some interval training? Short bursts of intense activity followed by recovery periods can be more manageable and just as beneficial when the heat is on.

Don't overlook the importance of flexibility. Summer is the perfect time for outdoor yoga sessions; a sunrise or sunset practice can be magical. The warmth helps muscles stretch further, minimizing the risk of injury. Find a class in the park, or roll out your mat in your own back garden—you'll connect with nature and enhance your flexibility in one delightful stroke.

Restorative activities are also paramount. Swimming is the quintessential summer exercise that cools your body while providing a full-body workout. It's gentle on the joints and an excellent way to recover from more intense activities. Kayaking, stand-up paddleboarding, and other water sports also blend adventure with exercise, ensuring your regimen remains enticing.

Adequate rest can't be overemphasized. It's the secret ingredient that lets your body heal and grow stronger. Factor in relaxation and leisure walks, especially on those balmy evenings. Use rest days to plan and prepare for more vigorous workouts or to simply soak up the tranquil summer vibes with mindfulness exercises in the great outdoors.

Hydration and sun protection are two hand-in-hand considerations for any summer regimen. Don't just drink water when you're thirsty; sip throughout the day. Supplement water intake with sports drinks that replace electrolytes lost through sweat on those scorching days. And never underestimate the sun—apply and reapply sunscreen, wear a hat, and opt for breathable, light-coloured clothing to reflect heat.

What about timing? Working out in the cooler parts of the day is more than just comfort; it's about safety. Dawn and dusk are ideal—bask in the pink hues of dawn or enjoy the respite offered by the evening's cooler air. Shifting workouts to these times mitigates the risk of heat exhaustion and allows for more intense sessions without battling midday heat.

Eat to fuel your summer activity. Fruits, vegetables, lean proteins, and whole grains will grant the energy needed for an active lifestyle while helping with recovery and hydration. Seasonal produce not only tastes better but can provide the nutrients your body craves during hotter months. Plus, it's always a good idea to plan meals around your workouts for optimal performance and recovery.

Balance also comes with progression. Begin with less demanding workouts to let your body acclimatize to the summer heat. Gradually increase intensity and duration as you build up a tolerance. It's better to underdo it initially than to overdo it and suffer from heat-related illnesses that can setback your exercise journey.

Don't forget to listen to your body's signals. Heat can exacerbate fatigue and make every step feel laborious. Adjust your activities accordingly. Sometimes, switching out a run for a walk or reducing the volume of exercise can be wiser choices. Being inflexible with your routine can lead to burnout or injury.

To keep the excitement alive, weave in some seasonal activities. Diversify your regimen with hiking, beach volleyball, or frisbee. Engaging in different forms of exercise will work new muscle groups and keep your mind engaged. Challenges don't have to be Everest-sized—small hills can provide great satisfaction too.

Lastly, keep an eye on air quality, particularly if you live in an urban area. Summer can bring about ozone alerts and higher pollution levels, which can impede breathing and overall health. Opt for indoor exercise or seek out greener areas during these times. Even an air-filtered mall walk can be a great fallback.

Building a holistic and balanced summer exercise regimen isn't just about pushing limits; it's about harmonizing with the season's pulse. A patient and measured approach that accommodates summer's heat will not only enhance your current fitness journey but set a sustainable pace for the seasons to come. Celebrate each stride under the sun, for summer's spirited dance is short-lived, and with each sunset, closer to its end.

It's about subtle readjustments, listening to the rhythm of the seasons, and allowing that cadence to dictate our movements. So here's to creating a regimen that's as fluid as a summer breeze and as revitalising as a dip in the ocean. Let's savour each glistening droplet of sweat as a testament to our commitment to well-being and the joy of immersing ourselves in the splendour of summer.

Chapter 4:
Autumn's Transition

As the heat of summer wanes and the lush greenery starts donning hues of amber and crimson, we're ushered into autumn – a season of transformation that reflects the very essence of change within us. Embracing the crisper air and the gentle fall of leaves isn't just poetic; it's a call to adapt our fitness routines to the magic enveloping the natural world. Think of autumn as nature's gentle nudge, encouraging us to swap the intensity of summer activities for routines that align with the cooler, introspective climate. The dimming daylight doesn't signal confinement indoors; rather, it's an invitation to witness the breathtaking palette only autumn can paint, the rustling leaves beneath our feet orchestrating a rhythm that motivates us even as the world slows down. As we jog through tree-lined paths or practise tai chi in dew-speckled parks, the air, scented with earth and rain, gifts our lungs a different kind of freshness, stirring an energy within that summer's scorch couldn't ignite. So let's lace up for the season of mellow fruitfulness, where every breath we take amidst the falling leaves deepens our connection to the earth and our very core.

Embracing Change: Adapting Workouts for Cooler Weather

As the flush of summer fades into the mosaic of autumn, it's not just the leaves that must transition. Our workouts, too, need to adapt to the nippier air and dwindling daylight. Cooler weather shouldn't cool our enthusiasm for outdoor exercise; rather, let's see it as an invitation to diversify our routines and challenge our bodies in new ways. After all, there's a certain invigoration that comes with a crisp jog amid the changing leaves or a brisk hike up a misty trail.

First things first: outfit yourself adequately. This means investing in layers that can be shed and donned as your body temperature fluctuates with exertion and rests. A moisture-wicking base layer, an insulating mid-layer, and a protective shell are your cool weather workout allies. With these, the chill won't stand a chance at damping your spirits or catching you with a post-workout shiver.

Switching up your workout times may also prove beneficial as we tilt away from the sun. Mornings are slower to warm up, which makes the midday sun, often a foe in the summer, a welcome friend in the cooler months. Plan your runs, walks, or rides for when the temperature peaks, and you'll soak in not just the warmth but likely some much-needed vitamin D, too.

If you're a pavement pounder, it's worth noting that the firmness of the ground changes with the temperature. Cooler weather can make surfaces more rigid, which means your joints might feel the difference. Consider migrating some of your runs onto trails with forgiving dirt or leaves, which can provide both a cushion and a visually stimulating course lined with autumnal glory.

Embrace strength training outdoors. Park benches double as dip stations, and children's play areas become jungle gyms for adults. Bodyweight exercises such as push-ups, pull-ups, and lunges adopt a fresh zest when done with a backdrop of the season's fiery palette. Plus, the cooler air can be much less stifling than the sticky heat, allowing you to push harder without the risk of overheating.

While you may have worked hard to acclimate to the heat of summer workouts, the body will soon need to adjust to internalize the cooler air. Breathing exercises can be particularly effective in this transition period. Use mindfulness to slow your breaths, take in the crisp air deeply, and let your body get accustomed to the change in temperature.

Moreover, this time of year offers unique activities that aren't always available in the summer - think about outdoor swimming in brisk waters or joining a local football or rugby club. The cold can enhance your endurance and make your heart pump more efficiently, making sports in cooler weather both a challenge and an invigorating experience. Don't forget, though, that warming up becomes even more crucial now to prevent pulls and strains.

Nature's gym isn't about locking into one activity; it's about utilising the elements and seasonally available surroundings. Autumn might be the perfect time to take up cycling when the roads are less sticky and busy with sun-seeking tourists. Or perhaps consider rowing to watch the scenery slide by on a reflective, foggy morning river. The water is usually calmer this time of year, making it ideal for beginners.

What about exploring new territories? Cooler weather often means fewer insects and less dense undergrowth, providing an excellent opportunity to uncover trails that were less friendly in the summer months. Leaf-covered paths provide new textures underfoot and the decreased foliage opens sight lines, offering fresh vistas and perspectives on familiar routes.

Some might find the dip in temperature a mental hurdle. Keeping a workout log can help you track not only your physical progress but also reflect on how the cooler conditions affect your overall well-being. Noting down those post-workout euphoric feelings can be motivating when the bed feels extra warm on a chilly morning.

Falling leaves aren't the only things to seize; take this chance to fall back in love with community events. Cooler weather often sees a resurgence in races and competitions: marathons, cycling tours, charity walks. These are not just opportunities to stretch your legs but also to immerse yourself in the communal spirit that often blossoms when people rally against the chill together.

And let's not forget the harvest season. Pre or post workout, the bounty of autumn's crops can enrich your meals with vitamins and antioxidants essential for recovery and energy. Plan your workouts around local orchards or farmer's markets, and treat yourself to seasonal goodies. Who says a brisk walk can't end with a fresh apple picked straight from the branch?

As the light fades earlier with each passing day, safety becomes paramount. Reflective clothing and headlamps should become mainstays in your evening workout attire. Taking precautions doesn't just ensure safety; it sets your mind at ease, allowing you to focus fully on the workout and the beauty enveloping you.

Yet, should the weather take a severe turn, be flexible. Adaptability is key to maintaining your fitness journey. Sometimes, cooler weather brings surprises like early snow or brittle ice. In such cases, it's wise to pivot to indoor workouts or exercises that can be performed safely at home. There's harmony in combining the vigour of outdoor exercises with the prudence of indoor practices.

Finally, stay inspired. Cooler weather casts a different light on nature, and its milder palette might reveal paths untraveled and landscapes unappreciated in the full sun of summer. Embrace this season's distinctive charm and let it fuel your workouts with a freshness akin to the brisk air you're learning to love.

Leaf-Peeping Fitness: Capitalising on Autumn Colours

Autumn arrives with a fanfare of crimson, gold, and fiery oranges, setting forests ablaze with colour. For the nature-loving fitness enthusiast, this season offers a unique window to take your workout into the glorious tableau of fall foliage. It's not just a feast for the eyes—there's something invigorating about the crisp air and the crunch of leaves underfoot that can rejuvenate your routine and bring a fresh perspective to your fitness goals.

The transformation of the landscape during autumn is more than mere scenery—it's a versatile backdrop for a myriad of outdoor activities that can enhance your physical well-being. Think trail running amidst a forest of golds and umbers, the uneven ground beneath your feet providing the perfect natural resistance to strengthen your legs and core. Or perhaps cycling through a park, the leaves forming a vibrant carpet on the path, their rustling your soundtrack for speed and endurance training.

It's also a season that invites you to slow down, to match the gentle descent of the leaves with mindful movements. Yoga in a quiet corner of a park, surrounded by amber and russet hues, can be both grounding and uplifting. Being present in such an environment allows you to connect deeply with your breath, your body, and the moment. It's not just exercise, it's a full-bodied experience that captivates all senses.

Strength training, too, can find a place among the autumn leaves. Park benches become your prop for step-ups and tricep dips. Tree trunks provide the perfect resistance for push-ups. And those fallen leaves? They make locating your hand and foot placements more challenging, thus engaging more muscles than the same movements might on a pristine gym floor.

Group activities gain an extra layer of appeal when they're set against a backdrop of fall foliage. Organizing a hiking or running group can be an excellent way to enjoy the beauty and companionship. These outings are not just opportunities for cardio; they are moments to share in the collective awe of nature's splendour, boosting your emotional health as well as your physical stamina.

But don't think you have to limit yourself to daylight hours. As the nights draw in, early evening jogs or walks offer a different experience of the autumn colours, with the softer light adding a different hue to the scenery. Headlamps or hand-held torches are, of course, essential as you navigate through the earlier nights, adding an element of adventure to your routine.

For those with a competitive spirit, autumn is ripe with races set against the most picturesque of canvases. Whether you're aiming to best your personal record in a 5k or simply want to run with friends, the extra motivation of a good cause and the vibrancy of the trail can propel you forward.

Nature's gym in autumn isn't just about physical exercise; it's a sensory journey. The rustle of leaves with every step, the visual dance of reds and yellows, and the scent of earthy decay meld to captivate and motivate. Perhaps it's the reminder of impermanence, the fleeting beauty of the season, that makes each workout feel more urgent, more vital.

One should not forget family fitness during this bountiful season. Scavenger hunts for different leaf types can be both an educational and physical activity as children dash from tree to tree, collecting their treasures. The more laid-back pace can be the perfect fit for family members of all ages, blending quality time with healthy habits.

Even on chillier days when you can see your breath in the air, the beauty of autumn dares you to step outside. Dressing in layers ensures comfort, allowing you to peel off or pile on as your body temperature adjusts to your exertion levels. Such preparation means there's seldom an excuse to miss the chance to engage with the outdoor gym autumn provides.

But what if the weather turns truly dreary? Even then, the multisensory aspect of leaf-peeping fitness offers a different kind of allure. Jogging through a light drizzle amidst the still-vivid foliage creates a refreshing contrast, a smile can't help but form as you feel like the sole inhabitant of a breathtaking, living watercolour painting.

As leaves continue to fall, navigating paths obscured by a thick carpet of foliage can add an element of unpredictability to your workouts. This natural obstacle course is not just fun; it fine-tunes your reflexes and heightens your awareness, beneficial skills for any fitness devotee.

And when the leaves have all but left their branches, don't think your leaf-peeping fitness must conclude. The bare skeletons of trees against an autumn sky can provide a stark, beautiful setting for reflection and meditation post-workout. The end of fall doesn't signify an end to outdoor fitness; rather, it's an invitation to witness yet another transition of nature's endless cycles.

In these months, as the world prepares to quieten for winter, embracing the kaleidoscope of autumn's colours in your fitness routine is to celebrate change. It's to move with the rhythms of the earth, to breathe in the transformation and to see it mirrored in your own physical and mental metamorphosis. So, lace up, step out, and let the crunch of leaves underfoot be the soundtrack to your autumn fitness journey.

Mindful Movement Amongst Falling Leaves

Pause for a moment and step outside. The air's cooler embrace signals the arrival of autumn, the season of transformation. Leaves adorned in fiery reds, warm oranges, and vibrant yellows begin their gentle descent towards Earth, creating a tapestry of colour that crunches underfoot. This isn't just a sight to behold; it's an open invitation to engage with nature through mindful movement. Whether you're watching leaves fall in a city park or a secluded forest, there's an undeniable charm that permeates this time of year and beckons you to move with awareness and serenity.

Autumn presents a unique opportunity to adapt your fitness routine to not only embrace the cooling temperatures but also to connect deeply with your surroundings. Mindfulness, the practice of being fully present and engaged in the moment, can be seamlessly integrated into outdoor exercises. As you journey through a landscape painted with the hues of fall, consider each step of your walk or run as a form of moving meditation.

Notice how the uneven terrain - a mosaic of leaves and earth - demands your attention, keeping you grounded in the present. The terrain offers a natural irregularity to your movement, enhancing your proprioception and engaging your core. As each leaf tumbles from the branch, you're reminded of nature's constant cycle of change and renewal, mirroring the changes you experience within your own body and mind as you engage in regular exercise.

When you incorporate mindfulness into your movement, you'll find a rhythm that syncs with the rustling leaves. Sync your breath with your stride, inhaling the crisp, cool air, and exhaling any tension. Feel your muscles engaging, your heart pumping, your body warming despite the chill, and notice the incredible machine that is your body working in perfect harmony with nature's symphony.

The act of moving amongst the falling leaves encourages a form of presence that might elude you on the treadmill or in the gym. Outdoor exercise during autumn can be an exquisite sensory journey. Allow your eyes to trace the dance of each leaf as it drifts to the ground, let your ears tune into the crunch beneath your feet, and breathe in the rich, earthy scent of decay that signifies rebirth in the natural world.

Vary your pace with the whims of the wind, which may gust and send a flurry of leaves skyward or may still, allowing a profound silence to envelope you. This is not just a workout; it's an interaction with the elements. There's a subtle beauty in synchronising your movements with the capricious nature of the breeze, ebbing and flowing just like the intensity of your exercise.

Yoga enthusiasts often find this time of year to be particularly enriching. Practising your asanas on a bed of leaves, the ground below supporting you as branches stretch above, brings a fresh perspective to your practice. Balancing poses become an even more focused endeavor as you stabilise on the soft and uneven surface.

For runners, the soft carpet of leaves can provide a respite for joints, offering a more forgiving surface than pavement or hard-packed dirt. Trail runners can relish the added challenge and joy of darting through a wooded landscape, the colours a moving blur as they pick their way through the natural obstacle course of roots and rocks.

Cycling through a forest path or down a city street lined with trees offers its own rewards. Feel the brisk air against your face and take in the fluctuating colours. Each pedal stroke feels purposeful, not just propelling you forward but keeping you attuned to the wonders passing by your handlebars.

Perhaps one of the simplest pleasures is hiking during the fall. The crunch underfoot, the muffled echo of wildlife preparing for winter, and the kaleidoscope of leaves falling around you can be almost hypnotic. Notice how your breath forms clouds in the cooler air, a visible reminder of your living, breathing connection with the environment.

While indulging in these mindful activities, the fall also presents an ideal moment to reflect on your physical progress. The year is waning, but your strength and perseverance are peaking. Each outdoor session is an opportunity to celebrate what your body has achieved and to set intentions for the coming winter months.

Remember to dress in layers when you're heading out for an autumnal workout. The air may be frigid at first, but your body will quickly heat up as you move. Keeping comfortable will only enhance your ability to stay present and revel in the sensory delicacies of the season.

Lastly, do not underestimate the value of stillness amidst the falling leaves. Take time to sit or stand in quiet contemplation, absorbing the abundant lessons autumn has to offer. This season, perhaps more than any other, has a way of whispering to us about impermanence, about letting go, and about the beauty to be found in both.

As you continue to visit nature's gym throughout the year, the changing scenery offers a plethora of experiences. Autumn's particular blend of crisp air, brilliant colours, and the constant motion of falling leaves provide a stunning backdrop for mindfulness and movement. Whether your preferred activity is running through golden-hued trails, cycling along winding paths, or stretching in the open air, fall's vibrant orchestra plays a tune of transformation for all who are eager to listen.

So, take a deep breath, lace up your shoes, and step out into the season of mindfulness and movement. Let it envelop you in its vibrant embrace as you find new ways to connect with yourself and the environment. This chapter isn't just about the dropping temperature or the changing colours. It's about dropping into the present moment and colouring your routine with the richness of autumnal fitness.

Chapter 5:
Winter's Wonderland

As the landscape transforms into a frost-kissed panorama, Winter's Wonderland beckons us with its unique allure, challenging our endurance and inspiring awe. There's something profoundly invigorating about crunching through fresh snow, feeling the bite of cold air on exposed cheeks, and watching one's breath spiral into misty clouds. Yet, it's more than just a picture-postcard scene; it's a playground that tests our physical limits and mental fortitude. The synchronicity of gliding on cross-country skis, the rhythmic dance of crackling ice beneath winter boots, and the joy that resonates from building snowmen, it's all available for those bold enough to step outside. So zip up your parka and cinch those snow boots, because embracing the icy embrace of winter not only heightens your fitness routine but also fortifies your resilience, making every warm sip of cocoa or snuggle by the fire a deserved slice of heaven. It's not just a season; for the adventurous spirit, it's a stage—one blanketed in snow and shrouded in the promise of tranquil solitude or boisterous snowball fights, if you're willing to make the first snow angel.

Cold Weather Resilience: Building Mental Toughness

Delving into the winter wonderland brings its unique challenges, stark beauty, and the need for a solid armoury of mental fortitude. Building mental toughness during the colder months isn't just about wearing the right thermal attire; it's about preparing your mind to both endure and embrace the drop in temperature and shortened days. Let's explore what it takes to cultivate a mindset that not only survives but thrives in the cold.

First and foremost, understanding the mental shift required for winter is critical. With less daylight and often more inclement weather, the mind can default to a state of resistance. It's in this space that you must find your stride. Start with small, manageable outdoor activities. As the fresh, crisp air hits your face, remind yourself that this sensation is not your adversary. It's the harbinger of invigoration, an awakening of your senses.

Set goals that are specific to winter. Whether it's mastering a new winter sport or improving your endurance in the cold, these objectives give you a laser focus that overshadows the discomfort. Track your progress. Each step in snow, each breath that turns to vapour before your eyes signifies your growing resilience.

Visualization is a powerful tool in your mental toughness toolkit. Picture yourself moving with ease across a frozen landscape, the cold a mere whisper against the backdrop of your determination. Regularly engaging in this practice can significantly alter your perception of the cold, framing it not as a hurdle but as a facilitator of strength.

Embrace the solitude winter often grants. The stillness of a snow-covered forest or a frosted city park lends itself to introspection. Use these quieter times to fortify your inner dialogue, turning thoughts of discomfort into affirmations of perseverance. "The cold is not my enemy, it's my challenge,"—repeat this as a mantra.

Preparation also plays a pivotal role. Equip yourself with the right knowledge of how the body reacts to cold conditions. Understanding the science of your body in winter aids in preventing unnecessary fears about what is normal when temperatures drop. An informed mind is a resilient one.

Mental toughness is also about adaptability. There might be days when a winter storm bars you from your planned run or hike. Rather than seeing it as a setback, adapt your routine indoors with high-intensity workouts or yoga sessions. See every change as a chance to grow and flex your mental adaptability muscles.

Nourish resilience from within—literally. The right nutrition can influence your mood and energy levels. Foods rich in vitamins and omega-3 fatty acids can boost your brain's serotonin levels, helping you combat the winter blues. Bring warmth from the inside out with hearty, nutritious meals that fuel both body and mind for cold weather exploits.

Another facet of building mental toughness is ensuring a community. While winter can sometimes isolify, seek out a tribe who loves the cold as much as you do, or perhaps even more. Together, you can push each other forward, share tips, and most importantly, validate each other's experiences. The power of a supportive community can't be overstated.

Sleep is another cornerstone of mental resilience. The longer nights of winter are your body's cue to rest and recover. Ensure you're getting quality sleep to cope effectively with the physical demands of cold weather activities. A well-rested mind is far better equipped to tackle the challenges of the season.

What's more, don't underestimate the impact of daylight on your mental well-being. Make the most of the daylight hours by syncing your outdoor activities to when the sun graces the sky. The infusion of natural light is not only essential for vitamin D synthesis but also uplifts your mood, fortifying your mental resilience against the cold.

When you're out braving the cold, focus on your breathing. The crisp winter air may feel sharp on the lungs initially, but deep, rhythmic breathing can help regulate your body's response to the cold.

Over time, this mindfulness in breathwork becomes a subconscious reflex, further bolstering your resolve.

Scaling up your winter experiences gradually is key. If you're new to cold-weather activities, don't rush into an arctic marathon straight away. Build your exposure slowly. Take note of how your body and mind adapt. These observations empower you, as you catalogue each victory over the cold, however small.

Lastly, remind yourself of the unique benefits the cold offers. The serene beauty of a landscape transformed by frost, the stillness that allows for clear thought, the exquisite contrast of a warm homecoming—these are treasures that only winter bestows. Reconceptualize the season not as an adversary, but as an exclusive backdrop for personal growth.

Winter can be a demanding coach, but the mental toughness garnered in its frosty domain is thoroughly transferable. The lessons learnt here seep into other areas of life, building a more resilient you, capable not just of withstanding but savouring the cold. Armed with these strategies, you can turn the darkest and coldest of seasons into a celebration of strength, stamina, and spiritual fortitude.

Indoor Versus Outdoor Training: The Winter Debate

As the frosty air settles and snow carpets the ground, the winter debate heats up amongst those dedicated to maintaining their fitness routines: to train indoors or brave the cold outdoors. It's a topic that stirs as much passion as a storm brewing over the horizon. But let's not reduce it to a simple either-or quandary; both indoor and outdoor training in winter have merits worth exploring.

Consider the cozy confines of a gym or your living room. It's enticing, isn't it? The warmth that hugs your skin, the predictability that comforts you—no gusty breezes or icy patches to disrupt your workout. Indoor training offers controlled temperatures, stability, and the convenience of equipment at arm's reach—excellent for maintaining fitness levels when the mercury drops. You can't quite beat the reliability of a treadmill run or a spin class when blizzards blitz the outside world.

Now, pivot your thoughts to the great outdoors. The crisp air invites you, chilly but invigorating, crisp, refreshing. Training outside in winter can be a soul-stirring experience. The landscape painterly in its monochrome palette, the silence of snowfall, the challenge of adapting to the elements—it's not just a workout; it's an adventure. It tests your mettle, pushes your boundaries, and rewards you with an undeniable sense of accomplishment.

But let's go beyond the idyllic. Outdoor winter training isn't just poetic; it's practical. It builds resilience. Your body adapts to the cold, learning to manage its core temperature, enhance circulation, and improve your overall immune response. The variance in terrain—whether it's snow, slush, or mud—strengthens your stabilising muscles, enhances your balance, and gives you a toughness that can't be replicated indoors.

What's more, exposing yourself to daylight, even the weak sunlight of shorter days, can bolster your vitamin D levels, stave off the winter blues, and maintain a circadian rhythm that indoor lighting can never quite mimic. For many, this is a critical tenet of mental health during the darker months.

Yet, we can't overlook the need for safety and sensibility. Outdoor training in the winter demands respect for the weather and its whims. We're talking about proper layering strategies, understanding hypothermia risks, and knowing when to call it a day. There's no heroism in risking frostbite or an injury due to a slip on unseen ice. The debate is moot if your wellbeing is compromised.

Indoor training, while safer on the surface, has its own set of considerations. Ventilation, especially in crowded gyms, is a concern during cold and flu season. Moreover, the monotony of indoor exercises can lead to a plateau in your progress and a decline in motivation. Breaking up the routine with occasional outdoor sessions might just bring back the spark needed to keep your fitness journey interesting and effective.

So, should you stick it out indoors or lace up for the great wintry outdoors? Perhaps the question is not which is better, but rather, how can you strategically combine the two? A blend of indoor and outdoor sessions could provide the balance between safety and exhilaration, comfort and challenge, monotony and diversity.

For those resistant to yielding to winters chill, the indoor route could be interspersed with brief outdoor endeavours. Think of brisk walks or short, high-intensity circuit workouts in your backyard or local park. Each burst of outdoor activity can serve as a reminder of nature's presence and a nudge to your resilience.

In contrast, the avid outdoor enthusiast might do well to occasionally step inside for workout sessions that require specific equipment or conditions not easily replicated outside. Weight training, certain types of yoga, and swimming, for instance, are generally better suited for the indoors, especially during the cold season.

Another perspective to adopt is periodisation—rotating the focus of your training with the seasons. Winter could be the perfect time to concentrate on building muscular strength indoors while maintaining cardiovascular endurance with outdoor runs or cross-country skiing.

And, of course, let's not forget the pure joy and childlike wonder that comes from winter outdoor activities: building a snowman, having a snowball fight, ice skating, or sledding. These aren't just fun and games; they're active, heart-healthy ways to engage with the cold that also bring along psychological uplift.

When decisions loom as heavy as a winter snowdrift, listen to your body and respect its cues. Balancing the enjoyment of your workouts with the need to stay healthy is key. On days when the cold bites a bit too fiercely, an indoor workout could be just what's needed. Conversely, when cabin fever sets in, a dose of outdoor training could be the antidote to restlessness.

In the end, the indoor versus outdoor training debate in winter mirrors the broader conversation about balance in our lives. Embrace the uniqueness of what each offers, and you'll find a harmonious rhythm to your fitness regimen that could only come with the changing seasons. This is not an ultimatum between two contrasting choices, but an invitation to dance with nature and adaptability, channelling the splendour and strength of winter into every step of your fitness journey.

Layering Strategies for Chilly Conditions

As the mercury dips and frost starts to glisten on the morning grass, outdoor enthusiasts face a conundrum: how to stay warm and dry without sacrificing mobility or comfort. It's a delicate balance, but with the right approach, you can conquer the cold and continue to enjoy the majesty of nature's winter composition.

The base layer is pivotal—it's the foundation upon which your cold-weather ensemble is built. Aim for materials that wick moisture away from your skin. That soggy sensation during chillier workouts is often the prelude to a deep chill once your pace slows. Synthetic fibers or merino wool excel in this, offering you a dry warmth that cotton just can't match. Plus, merino wool has a knack for countering unpleasant odours, an attribute that's much appreciated during lengthy excursions in the outdoors.

Next, let's add some more insulation. The middle layer's mission is to trap warmth, and here, fleece or a lightweight synthetic insulation reigns supreme. They trap air close to your body, forming a thermal buffer against the winter's nip. Furthermore, they are generally breathable, ensuring that you don't overheat when your endeavours intensify.

Consider your outer layer the guardian against the elements. It's a tough job, fending off biting winds and deflecting rain or snow. Look for an outer shell that's waterproof yet breathable, a barrier that can hold its own against the most curmudgeonly of climes without turning you into a walking sauna.

Don't neglect your extremities. Head, hands, and feet are notorious for succumbing to the cold. A good hat will conserve crucial heat that bids farewell from your head, while gloves should be insulated but not so bulky that they compromise dexterity. Socks should echo the ethos of your base layer—comfortable, warm, and moisture-wicking.

Layering doesn't end with fabric. Air is a remarkable insulator. Ensure your layers allow for a cushion of air between them, and you'll find warmth in even the most reluctant of temperatures. And in the spirit of flexibility, embrace zippered garments or those with vents. When the sun graces you with its presence, or your activity peaks, you'll appreciate the quick reprieve they provide. Merely unzip and let your body breathe.

Modularity is your trusty companion in the great outdoors. Select garments that seamlessly integrate, so you can add or peel layers without a hitch. This approach empowers you to adapt to the day's narrative, adding a whisper of warmth when the plot thickens or unfurling your outfit as the tension wanes.

A common blunder is overdressing, leading to a sweltering experience that can culminate in a rapid cooldown once you stop moving. Start off feeling slightly cool, knowing your body will generate heat as you persevere along the path. Trust in your planning and your body's intrinsic ability to regulate its temperature.

When precipitation makes an unscheduled cameo, your preparation shines. Swiftly adjust layers to meet the aqueous challenge. A wet body can quickly become a cold body, so ensuring you stay dry under that waterproof shell is crucial. Stow an extra layer in a dry bag, just in case the skies decide to pour their heart out.

Embrace layering as a dynamic process, much like the landscapes you traverse. Conditions fluctuate, and so too should your attire. Approach layering with both foresight and a degree of improvisation, ready to adapt to the whispers of the wind or the chill embrace of the cloud cover.

But layering isn't merely a practical measure—it's a ritual that aligns you with the rhythms of nature. Each layer is a stanza in your outdoor ode; they compose a dialogue between your body and the elements. Tune in to the chill of the air, the warmth of your breath, the snug embrace of your gear—each sensation is part of the symphony of outdoor serenity.

As dusk heralds the day's close and temperatures commence their descent, another layer, this time a lightweight insulated jacket, might find its purpose. Stopping for a breather or setting camp as the light mounts its final defense against night's advance—those are the moments when an extra layer makes all the difference.

Finally, consider the longevity of your apparel. Invest in quality that endures across seasons, pieces that stand the test of time. The love for the outdoors is perennial, and so your gear should be built to match that ceaseless zeal.

And when the chill really sets in, remember that movement is warmth. Nature's gym is all about staying mobile, so keep pace, maintain intensity, and let your layered fortress do the rest.

So there it is, the art of layering for the chilly conditions that winter brings. Embrace it as you embrace the cold—wholeheartedly and without reservation. Stay warm, stay dry, and above all, stay in motion. It's the dance of layer upon layer that lets you stride with confidence into the embrace of winter's wonderland.

Chapter 6:
Rain or Shine: Adapting to Wet Weather

As we transcend the crisp embrace of winter's touch, we find ourselves peering into the cloud-laden skies of damper days. Here in Chapter 6, it's time we tackle the droplets and drizzles head-on. Don't let a bit of rainfall dampen your spirits or curtail your expedition into Nature's Gym. There's a certain charm to the rhythm of raindrops as they pitter-patter against the canopy of leaves above, transforming trails into a glistening wonderland. Embrace the slick, wet earth beneath your feet; it's an open invitation to fine-tune your balance and strengthen your core. We're going to learn how to clad ourselves with the right attire that repels water while still allowing our skin to breathe—because, after all, getting soaked to the bone isn't the aim of the game. It's all about adapting our routines, not just to endure but to relish the wet weather workouts, allowing that fresh, petrichor-scented air to invigorate our souls as we splash through puddles, our faces beaming with a childlike joy. Rain or shine, nature beckons us to confront its elements with zest, and in doing so, we unlock a dimension of fitness that's as liberating as it is empowering. So pull on your waterproof boots and let the rain caress your face because it's just another facet of nature waiting to be experienced in its full, life-affirming glory.

Rainproof Routines: Staying Dry and Comfortable

As we delve deeper into a lifestyle that embraces outdoor activity irrespective of the whims of the weather, addressing the occasional, inevitable drizzle or the sometimes relentless rain becomes essential. Let's face it: getting soaked is a thrill for some, but staying dry and comfortable can often keep morale higher and prevent the damp squib scenario of abandoned workouts due to misjudged weather.

The cornerstone of any plan to withstand the wet is your clothing. It's not just about waterproofs; consider the layers that sit comfortably beneath, ensuring they are crafted from moisture-wicking fabrics. Remember, a skin not stifling in its own sweat is one that can relish the rain rather than resent it. This isn't just about comfort; it's also a nod to maintaining body temperature and making sure that physical performance isn't hindered by soggy attire.

Now, let's talk about those rain jackets. They aren't just a shield against rain; they're your armour in maintaining enthusiasm when the skies open up. A good waterproof jacket is breathable and lightweight, making it the go-to option. Sure, there are times when the heavens pour liberally, but a breathable waterproof ensures you won't be cooking in a self-made sauna.

Don't overlook the importance of a decent hat. It keeps the rain off your face, helps maintain visibility, and prevents waterlogging your mood. In a deluge, your sight beneath a hood is as trustworthy as your commitment to step out the door – so invest in a brim that keeps the rain off your specs or lashes.

Speaking of vision, if you wear glasses, there's nothing more trying than a blurred view mid-jog. Anti-fog sprays can be a spectacle-wearer's best friend in the rain. This extra step before you step out can mean the difference between a serene run and a soggy struggle.

In considering lower body attire, waterproof trousers or running tights with water-resistant properties can make strides a lot more inviting. If trousers seem too cumbersome, consider water-resistant spray for your regular leggings or tights. It's these little hacks that keep the routine rolling, even when the clouds are uncooperative.

When it comes to your feet, soggy socks can transform an empowering exercise into a trudge of desperation. Waterproof shoes or at least ones with a decent level of water resistance are a wise choice. And if you can't sidestep a puddle, ensure your socks can. Wick away moisture with a pair that keeps your toes as dry as possible.

Understandably, the monsoon-esque weather might not summon a surge of enthusiasm for a workout. But having a rain cape or packable poncho can pack a punch for such days. They're easy to stow away and simple to drape over during unexpected downpours, keeping your resolve as undampened as your attire.

Gloves are often an afterthought until numbed fingers remind us of their necessity. In rain, opt for lightweight, water-resistant gloves. While they might not keep out a torrent, they'll fend off enough to keep the digits happy and functional. After all, what use are hands if they can't grip on a rainy run or outdoor gym session?

Let's not forget the flora and fauna – while you're out there marvelling at rain-washed nature, ensure you don't disturb it with a cacophony of crinkling. Choose rain gear that's mindful of the soundscape; soft, rustle-free fabrics contribute to a harmonious outing and let you remain part of the ambience rather than an interruption to it.

Stacking up on waterproof gear is all well and good, but it's vital not to be weighed down. Lightweight is the watchword here. Your waterproof ensemble should enable freedom of movement, not restrict it. This holds especially true for backpacks, which should be compact, fitted with a rain cover, and not turn into a sodden burden.

Remember: the right mindset is part of your kit. When you embrace the weather rather than brace against it, you unlock a level of freedom. Shed the dread of the downpour and view each droplet as a part of your path to resilience. After all, a little water is simply nature's way of cheering you on.

Maintaining dryness isn't solely a quest for the right clothing; it's about how you engage with the environment. Seek out sheltered routes when appropriate: a canopy of trees, for instance, can and will offer a reprieve from the elements, allowing you to catch your breath without catching a cold.

Finally, your routine itself may need tweaking in the rain. Adjusting your expectations and perhaps lowering the intensity can prevent injuries on slippery surfaces. It's about being prudent, not hesitant; swap that trail run for a road route if stability is in question, or that high-intensity boot camp for a bodyweight circuit under some shelter.

Wrapping up your rain-resistant regimen, it's about finishing as you started: dry and upbeat. Planning your return into a warm, dry space helps your mind stay focused and your body, grateful. Post-workout, invest in quick-drying towels and a dry change of clothes to lock in that sense of accomplishment, rather than dampness.

In essence, rainproof routines are more than a practicality; they're a badge of honour, a statement that says you're undeterred and unswayed by the storms, literal or metaphorical. Each drop of rain is a reminder of your commitment to wellbeing, stability in the face of instability, and joy in what nature offers, regardless of its moods.

Puddle-Splashing to Fitness: Embracing the Wet

Think of that sensation as a child, when jumping into a puddle wasn't met with a scolding, but with the joyous abandon of carefree play. Now, let's transition that ethos into the realm of fitness, where the drizzle and downpour aren't deterrents but invigorating challenges. Embracing a soaking landscape isn't about defiance, but about thrills and the countless health benefits that accrue when you merge an open mindset with outdoor workouts, regardless of a bit of rain.

There is undeniable magic in the atmosphere post-rainfall. The air is crisp, revitalised and filled with the fresh scent of petrichor. Setting out for a jog on dampened paths, you'll be surprised by the increase in your sensory awareness. The wet conditions heighten your focus and connection to your surroundings, leading to a more mindful approach to exercise.

Admittedly, some may balk at the idea of venturing out into the wet. Yet, it's worth realising that rain can significantly intensify your workout. The resistance of water adds a beneficial layer of difficulty to each movement. Each step in a saturated field, each push against the surging currents of a rain-swollen river in your kayak, they all require more effort, more energy, hence boosting your endurance and strength over time.

Another aspect of puddle-splashing workouts is its inherent unpredictability. The slick terrain forces your muscles to work differently, to stabilise, adjust, and react spontaneously. This not only builds physical agility but mental acuity as well. It can be particularly beneficial for improving balance and coordination, essential skills that transfer across numerous athletic disciplines.

Naturally, wet conditions are a boon for cooling down your body during intense sessions. The precipitation can help in regulating your body temperature, enabling you to workout for longer periods without feeling as overwhelmed by heat as in dry conditions. Plus, let's be honest, who doesn't love the feeling of rain gently pelting down, working as nature's own cooling system?

Of course, equipping oneself with the proper gear is essential, as detailed in our spring all-weather gear guide. Waterproof attire not only protects you from getting soaked to the bone but also brings practicality and comfort to your routines, allowing for freedom of movement and the confidence to immerse yourself—that's right, even lie down in a puddle for those crunches or yoga poses!

Now consider the unique workout opportunity that puddles present. Case in point: plyometrics. The splashy exits and entries from a puddle during jump squats or hops add a layer of resistance and fun. The water's unpredictability requires more power, thus intensifying the workout and, importantly, the splash element makes it enjoyable and playful, which leads to a better relationship with exercise.

While water adds resistance, it also provides a therapeutic aspect. Hydrotherapy, which uses water's unique properties for pain relief and treatment, is an established concept. While not entirely equivalent, working out in puddles or gentle streams can offer a massaging effect on the muscles, with the added bonus of natural, fresh water.

Engaging in wet weather enriches not only your physical capabilities but your psychological resilience. Many shy away from a downpour, but embracing it head-on reinforces a mindset of adaptability and robustness. You'll nurture a sense of accomplishment that's unique to conquering the rain, proving to yourself that your commitment to fitness isn't water-soluble.

Let's also acknowledge the softer, more serene benefits. Rainfall has a rhythm, a cadence that can synchronise with your motions. Similar to the calming effect of a white noise machine, rain has the ability to create a bubble of focus and calm around you, making it a surprisingly meditative environment to train in.

Children, they have it right, don't they? Their instinctual gravitation towards puddles can be a reminder for us all. To embrace the wet is to connect with a primal joy of being in nature, to shake off societal inhibitions, and to literally make a splash. It's an invitation to play and to affirm that fitness can be fun, whatever the weather.

Moreover, variety is the spice of life—and of fitness routines. For those used to indoor gyms or dry outdoor trails, a rain-drenched workout can be a refreshing change of pace. And embracing such variety is beneficial not just for the body, but for the mind, keeping your routine from stagnating.

And let's not overlook the sociability factor. Group workouts in the rain can be a bonding experience like no other. There's a sense of solidarity in facing the elements together, which can foster stronger connections within workout communities. Shared laughter at shaking off water like a group of friendly dogs after a rainstorm can't be discounted for its uplifting effects.

In conclusion, puddle-splashing to fitness isn't merely about exercise. It's about dissolving barriers, both physical and mental. It's an exercise in joy, pushing boundaries, and embracing every droplet life throws your way. So, next time the clouds gather and the skies open, don that waterproof gear, find your nearest puddle, and leap into an enthralling workout that will rejuvenate your body, and perhaps more significantly, your spirit.

And remember, the weather never truly dictates the ability to pursue fitness—it simply provides a variety of stages and backgrounds for your journey. Every puddle you splash through is a testament to your commitment, a dynamic dance step in the choreography of outdoor training, and a celebration of nature's unpredictable yet wholly invigorating splendor.

Chapter 7:
Wind's Dynamic Resistance

As we emerge from the ebb and flow of rain-soaked workouts discussed in the previous chapter, it's time to turn our attention skyward to the capricious dance of the wind and its role in shaping our outdoor pursuits. In 'Wind's Dynamic Resistance', the unseen currents become a potent symbol of nature's paradox: both a challenging adversary and a powerful ally. We'll learn to read the air's mood and flow with its rhythm, for it's in this breezy ballet that we discover resistance doesn't cease our efforts; it refines them. Think of the resistance as not just a barrier but as nature's own dynamic gym apparatus, ready to push you further, make you stronger, and, interestingly enough, propel you in directions you might not have otherwise taken. Let's navigate through the gusts and lulls, harnessing the wind's energy to add an invigorating twist to our outbound exercise, while knowing when to lean in and when to let the kite of our ambition soar on the breeze.

Harnessing the Breeze: Kite Running and More

If you've not yet felt the tug of a kite string in a brisk wind, you're missing out on an exhilarating connect with the skies. Kite running isn't just for kids; it's an absolute wonder for folks looking to spice up their outdoor routines. The wind, that unpredictable force of nature, becomes your dance partner—and what a magnificent partner it is.

Kite running is much more than just sprinting with a colourful tail in tow; it's about agility, coordination, and the sheer joy of movement.

Imagine this: an open field, the breeze gently caressing the treetops, and you with a kite in hand, poised to harness the wind. There's the initial thrill as the kite lifts into the air, and then the steady challenge of keeping it aloft. Sometimes it dips and dives unpredictably, urging you to sprint, twist, turn, and leap. Your body naturally syncs with the rhythms of the wind, engaging muscles you didn't even know you had. It's a full-body workout, disguised as child's play.

Here's the thing—the benefits go beyond the physical. There's a meditative quality to kite flying that sharpens the mind. You have to read subtle shifts in the breeze, adjust your movements, maintain concentration. It's a practice in mindfulness that can leave you feeling refreshed and invigorated, mentally clear and focused.

But let's expand the canvas. Kite running is just the beginning. There's kite surfing for those who crave the rush of the surf and the challenge of balancing on a board while controlling a powerful kite above. Kite buggying offers a blend of land sailing and flying, delivering an adrenaline spike as you steer a three-wheeled cart powered by nothing but the wind. These activities don't just make the outdoors your gym—they make it your playground.

Of course, approach these wind-driven pursuits with respect. The same breeze that grants you wings can be capricious. Invest time in understanding the nuances of your chosen activity and the environmental cues. Safety is paramount—proper gear, knowledge of the wind patterns, and sometimes the presence of an instructor are essential elements to ensure a fun and safe experience.

Let's not forget about the social aspect. While kite running can be a solitary venture, it often draws curious onlookers and fellow enthusiasts. It can quickly turn into a social event, where tips are swapped, styles are compared, and friendships are formed. A sunny weekend in the park with kites dotting the sky can be a vibrant community-building exercise

For the family-oriented amongst us, introducing children to the wonders of the wind can be a gratifying experience. They'll learn about aerodynamics, the environment, and the nuances of weather, all while engaging in a healthy dose of outdoor exercise. It's a way to teach kids the value of persistence and guide them through the failures and triumphs of watching a kite soar.

And it's not just a daylight affair. For those intrigued by the night, imagine flying a kite under a blanket of stars, led lights illuminating the canvas against the dark sky—an otherworldly experience that brings a touch of magic to your fitness regimen.

Dive deeper, and you'll find that the world of kite flying is steeped in rich cultural history. Different cultures have their unique kite designs and traditions, and kite festivals are held worldwide where the sky bursts into life with elaborate shapes and colors. It's a glorious celebration of the wind and its place in our heritage.

Still, wind-based activities aren't completely without environmental consideration. As responsible enthusiasts, it's on us to pick up after ourselves, use sustainable materials, and educate others on preserving the natural settings we so deeply enjoy. It's all part of the give-and-take of enjoying the great outdoors.

So next time the breeze stirs and you feel that itch for an outdoor exploit, consider kite flying in its various forms. Whether you choose to keep your feet planted firmly on the ground or take to the waves or sands, there's something undeniably compelling about taming and cooperating with the energy of the wind.

There's a final important note on preparation before you embark on your wind-powered journey—check the local weather and wind conditions. Understand the best times for your adventure, and make sure to gear up accordingly. This information is crucial for both safety and enjoyment.

In conclusion, there's a wonderful world of wind out there waiting for you. Kite running and its sibling activities present boundless opportunities to engage with nature, rejuvenate the spirit, and enliven the body. They encourage us to look to the skies—not as distant, unreachable expanses, but as integral parts of our outdoor gym. So, go on, harness that breeze and let it propel you into new realms of fitness and joy.

Wind's Challenges and Advantages: A Balancing Act

The whisper and roar of the wind are as intrinsic to the outdoor experience as the earth beneath our feet and the sky above our heads. It's a force that's ever-present, whether we notice its gentle caress or brace against its formidable gales. Let's delve into the complexities of this enigmatic element, exploring both the trials and boons it presents to our physical activities and mental fortitude.

The challenges set forth by the wind are immediate and palpable. If you've ever cycled headfirst into a strong wind, you know it's like tackling an invisible hill. This added resistance demands more from your muscles and your heart, turning what might have been an easy ride into an unexpected workout. It's not just about physical strain, though. The wind can chill you to the bone, carry your words away before they reach a companion's ears, and it can dispirit you if you're not prepared for its relentless push.

Yet, in this challenge lies an untapped advantage. The resistance we battle can be the resistance we seek. Just as weightlifters need the gravity that makes the barbell heavy, those who embrace outdoor activities can use the wind's might to strengthen their resolve and power. Runners find their strides in the buffeting gusts, bikers become more robust, rowers fight a tangible opponent, and each breath becomes a measure of the strength you gain in the face of adversity.

Beyond the physical, wind engages the mind and demands a strategic approach. You'll learn the art of angling your body to slice through the air, of finding paths shielded by trees or buildings, of employing tactics that sailors know well — sometimes you tack with the wind to reach your destination, even if it's not a straight line.

Let's switch gears and consider the gentler side. A light breeze can be the companion that cools your skin under a high sun, that fills your lungs with clean air, that dances with you as you dash through the open wilderness. It's refreshing, an ally that wards off overheating and revitalises your spirits. Herein the wind can be a friend, making a summer's jog an absolute delight.

Wind also heightens our senses. In its presence, you're more aware of your surroundings, your body's movements, and your connection to the environment. It brings the scents of far-off places, whispering tales of lands you've yet to see. It rustles leaves, creates waves, and joins the chorus of nature's soundscape.

What's more, engaging with the wind can enhance our mental resilience. Outdoor enthusiasts who routinely challenge the wind know this well — there's a metaphor to be found in standing firm against the gusts or using its force to propel you forward. It's a practice of patience and perseverance, teaching us about adaptation and acceptance.

And let's not overlook the pure exhilaration that comes with certain wind-powered sports. Kitesurfing, sailing, windsurfing — there's something inherently liberating about harnessing this natural force to skate across water or soar through the sky. The wind is both an obstacle and an engine, and those who understand its nuances can find joy in its dynamic embrace.

However, wind also brings unpredictability. It can change suddenly, shift directions without warning, and transform from friend to foe in moments. This unpredictability keeps us alert and engaged, but it also teaches us to be prepared and adaptive, to respect nature's whims and to always have a plan B when venturing out into the open air.

Moreover, wind has the uncanny ability to make us feel small, humbling us with its vast power. But in this humility, there's a profound lesson about our place in the greater scheme of things — it encourages gratitude for the shelter of our homes and an appreciation of the forces that shape our world.

In conclusion, engaging with the wind is indeed a balancing act. It's about embracing the struggle and finding the subtle currents that aid your journey. It's about the mental dance between frustration and elation, between fight and flight, between resistance and surrender. As you step outside and feel the breeze or the bluster, know that each gust has a lesson to teach and a strength to impart, if only we're willing to lean in or let go.

So next time the wind rises, whether you're setting out on a trek, clipping into your bike pedals, or unrolling your yoga mat in the park, consider what the wind brings to the table. Not just as another weather condition to dress for but as an active participant in your outdoor endeavour. It might just change the way you perceive the world around you — full of energy, constantly in motion, and always inviting you to play.

The wind can be mercurial, but that too has its purpose. As outdoor enthusiasts, we learn to embrace the capricious nature of the wind and, indeed, the world. It's part of the adventure, of what makes our activities not just a physical pursuit but a full-sensory experience. It's all about finding harmony in the chaos, peace in the disturbance, and joy in every breath of air.

So, when you engage with the wind, remember: it's a force to be reckoned with, offering both resistance and support, challenge and opportunity. It's a component of our environment that demands respect, preparation, and understanding. But it also provides a playground for strength, skill, and spiritedness. Navigate wisely, and you'll discover that the wind, with all its moods, is a most profound teacher.

Chapter 8:
Snow and Ice: Extreme Elements

As the last leaves bid their silhouetted farewell and the landscape dons its frosty coat, embracing winter's chill becomes not just a possibility, but a thrilling adventure. Snow and ice transform the ordinary into a playground for persistence and daring; they become the ultimate test of grit. Believe me, there's nothing quite like the rush of carving a path through untouched powder or the victorious battle against the slip of underfoot ice. It demands resilience and wit—qualities you can't help but cultivate out in winter's grasp. This chapter is all about facing these extreme elements head-on, learning to revel in the crunch beneath your boots, the sculptural beauty of frost, and the brisk air that makes every breath a defiant act against the sluggish comfort of the indoors. We'll prep for anything from an impromptu snowball fight to an intentional snowshoe hike, ensuring each icy encounter isn't just endured, but zealously enjoyed. So layer up, it's time to challenge the silent, snowy sentinels of winter—they're inviting you to dance.

Snow Sports and Activities: Beyond the Basics

Shifting our focus to a winter playground, we realise that the potential for thrill and personal challenge doesn't freeze with the water. Once you've mastered the beginner slopes and the art of staying upright on skis or a snowboard, an entire mountain range of possibilities beckons. Let's carve a path through the more advanced territories of snow sports, where we can ramp up our skills, find new thrills and even mix fitness with creativity in the snow.

First, consider backcountry skiing and splitboarding—a test of endurance as much as it is a descent into pure freeriding bliss. Venturing off the groomed paths calls for a heightened level of awareness and an appreciation for the serenity that ungroomed wilderness provides. But with this freedom comes the responsibility of understanding the terrain, the weather patterns, and the need for avalanche safety knowledge. The silence as you ascend, save for the crunch of snow underfoot, becomes a meditative practice before the exhilarating descent.

If the silent swoosh of skis isn't quite your tempo, you might take to the pulsating rhythm of snowmobiling. It's power at your fingertips, but with that power comes the need for control and respect for the machine—and the landscape. Each twist and turn introduces new challenges: from navigating hidden obstacles to reading the snow's consistency. And when done too recklessly, it can wreak havoc on pristine environments.

Now let's pivot—literally, for those about to learn—towards ice skating. Not just in circles at your local rink but out on a frozen lake where the vast expanse invites a dance with nature. Glide and spin, feeling the crisp air as your partner, in a ballet of balance and flow. But remember, safety checks are key before stepping onto wild ice; a serene surface doesn't always guarantee solidity.

Snowshoeing, with its roots in ancient survival, today presents a slower-paced, soul-soothing way to explore and connect with the snow-enshrouded landscapes. With today's lightweight equipment, there's no feeling quite like floating atop deep snow, where each step is an imprint on a vast white canvas. As you delve into remote areas, the tranquillity might just whisper the secrets of winter wildlife, otherwise unseen.

Adventure seekers might find their call in ice climbing: A vertical ascent against shimmering walls that demands precision, strength, and respect for the ever-changing ice. The clink of ice axes and crunch of crampons become a unique symphony, heralding your progress. It's a physical dialogue between you and the frozen cascade, each movement deliberate, every hold a triumph of will.

And then there's cross-country skiing, a test of endurance and poise, offering a heart-pumping traverse across miles of frosted terrain. Unlike its downhill cousin, here the joy comes from the journey itself; it's about rhythm, technique, and the satisfaction of each push travelling miles of wilderness trails that slice through silent forests and over frozen brooks.

For something less conventional, have you considered building a snow sculpture or ice art? It's about seeing the potential in a mound of snow, crafting and chiselling until your imagination takes a chill form. It's playful, yet it can be an all-consuming workout, as anyone who has wrestled with a snowdrift or ice block knows well.

Team sports don't take a break in winter, either. Ice hockey and curling provide a community experience that can simultaneously light up competitive fires and stoke the spirit of camaraderie. The clatter of sticks, the roar of a stone across the ice – these sounds encapsulate the essence of winter team sports, demanding tactical play, physical prowess and sharp precision.

Biathlon, combining the calm precision of rifle shooting with the intense physical demand of cross-country skiing, introduces a compelling twist to winter sports. It requires mastering the art of swiftly switching between relentless motion and the stillness necessary for accurate marksmanship. The twofold challenge demands a steely focus and the capability to transition smoothly between contrasting states of physical exertion.

Moving beyond traditional sports, winter allows for the innovation of new hybrid activities. Ever heard of snowkiting? Imagine harnessing the wind to glide across snow and ice on a board or skis, adding a whole different dimension to winter sports—part sailing, part flying, and pure exhilaration.

Moreover, dog sledding offers a unique blend of adventure and heritage, drawing you into an ancient pact with canines. The patter of paws against snow, the breathless rush of cold air, and the primal connection between human and dog awaken a primal joy and a unique form of partnership-based teamwork.

Another engaging sport that's flown under the radar for many is ski joëring, where skiers are pulled by horses, dogs, or even motor vehicles. It offers a quirky blend of skiing skills and the trust in your animal or mechanical partner, resulting in a heart-pumping synergy of speed and exhilaration right at the intersection of tradition and modernity.

But winter activities aren't all about high adrenaline. Take a long-distance sledding trip, where the art of packing, navigation and winter camping skills are as essential as the physical work of sledding. It redefines the concept of journey, presenting the wilderness not as a space to conquer, but as a companion to respect and understand.

The realm of snow and ice, as we've seen, is far from barren; it's a fertile field for the adventurer, the artist, and the athlete in us all. Fostering a relationship with this cold yet captivating environment is not just about chasing adrenaline but about discovering new rhythms, perspectives, and feelings of aliveness. As you embrace these advanced winter activities, remember they're more than thrills; they're opportunities to grow, to learn, and to resonate deeply with the silent poetry of winter.

Safe Practice in Slippery Situations

Imagine a pristine blanket of snow, a sleek sheen of ice, or a road slicked by melting frost. The allure is undeniable—nature cloaked in its wintry finery beckons you to step out and embrace the chill. However, venturing out into the frosty realm is not devoid of its perils. The key to thriving in these conditions is a mix of preparation, awareness, and respect for the ever-changing elements.

Let's first consider footwear, which is arguably your most crucial ally against the whims of slippery terrain. Traction is paramount. Opt for shoes with grippy soles designed for icy conditions or consider attachments like crampons or spikes that can be fixed onto your regular boots or trainers for that extra grip. After all, slipping is no laughing matter when a single fall could result in an injury that keeps you indoors for weeks.

Balance and gait come next. When you're venturing across ice or slippery surfaces, adjustments to your usual posture and movements are in order. Keep your centre of gravity over your feet by taking shorter, more deliberate steps—akin to a penguin's waddle, if you will. This isn't a fashion parade; it's about keeping upright and progressing safely.

Should you encounter a particularly slick patch, refrain from panicking. Avoid sharp, quick movements. It can be helpful to soften your knees and use your arms for balance. Let's not underestimate the power of arm movement—swinging them in coordination with your steps can do wonders for maintaining your balance.

If you've fallen before, you know the instinctive response is to stiffen up. Contrary to that impulse, it's essential to try and relax your body if you're going down. A loose body is less prone to serious injury. Teach yourself to fall sideways rather than backwards to avoid tailbone or head injuries. And remember, this is about minimizing harm, not evading the inevitable bruises that come with winter's touch.

Next on the agenda is the need to be visible. Shorter days and inclement weather can reduce visibility. Reflective clothing and lights are not just accessories; they're necessities that can mean the difference between being seen and an unwelcome encounter with a cyclist or motorist who didn't notice you until too late.

When it's cold, your muscles will require more time to warm up before they're ready for exertion. Spend a little extra time on your warm-up routine to get your blood pumping and your muscles limber. This isn't just about comfort; warm muscles are far less likely to sprain or strain than cold ones.

While moving through snowy terrains, stay aware of the risk of ice lurking beneath the snow's surface. Trudging in fresh snow can offer better grip than a path that has been compacted by many feet. It might be harder work, but it's often safer. And there's a primal pleasure in being the first to leave your footprints in fresh snowfall—indelible proof of your passage through winter's stillness.

Also, let's spare a thought for hydration. The winter air, brutally cold as it may be, can actually be quite dry. Don't be deceived by the lack of sweat; your body is still losing water through breathing and the dryness of the air. Keep sipping water—it's just as crucial as during a summer's day.

Moreover, pay attention to weather warnings and be flexible in your plans. A sudden drop in temperature overnight can turn that familiar jogging path into an ice rink. Changing your route or postponing your exercise session in extreme conditions is a wise move. Nature is a majestic force, but it's one that commands respect and can humble even the most experienced amongst us.

We mustn't forget about layering either. Dress warmly in layers that can be easily removed or added. Your body will warm up as you exercise, so having layers to adjust to your comfort level will prevent sweating—which, paradoxically, can make you even colder as moisture saps your body's warmth.

If you're venturing into these frosty realms often, consider learning some basic first aid. Understanding how to treat minor injuries like sprains or recognizing signs of frostbite and hypothermia may not only help you but could be invaluable in assisting others who might be in distress.

For those particularly hazardous days, consider indoor alternatives. A treadmill facing a window or winter sports simulation classes can provide a satisfactory substitute for the real deal until conditions improve. And on that note, some practices are inherently risky on ice—high-speed cycling, for one—give them a skip unless you're specially equipped and experienced in these conditions.

Accompanying someone experienced or in a small group can offer both moral support and additional safety. There's comfort in numbers, and assistance is immediately available if someone should take a tumble. Plus, shared experiences, even challenging ones, tend to create lasting bonds and stories that'll warm you for seasons to come.

Finally, always let someone know where you're going and when to expect you back. Remote areas that are peaceful in good weather can quickly turn into dangerous territory when the weather shifts. A communication plan can be your lifeline in unexpected circumstances. It's a simple step, but its importance can't be overstated.

With these considerations firmly in mind, the icy outdoors transforms from a treacherous beast to an exhilarating playground. Patience, preparation, and a hearty dose of caution can enable you to dance across the slippery stage of winter with confidence and, dare I say, even a bit of panache. And isn't that blend of safety and adventure what draws us to nature's gym in every season?

Cold-Climate Conditioning whispers promises of breathtaking landscapes glazed in white, challenges that sculpt not only the body but the will, and the pure joy of visible breaths in crisp air. It is in this wintry realm that nature chisels its most resolute athletes. Training in the cold is an art; a delicate balance between respecting the elements and harnessing them to forge fortitude within us.

Begin by acknowledging the bite of the cold—it is not an adversary but a companion in your fitness journey. You can condition your body to withstand and even relish the frost, turning every shiver into a step towards steadfast endurance. Before embarking on your first snowy run or ice-clad hike, take the time to acclimate. Your body needs to transition from indoor warmth to the bracing outdoor chill gradually.

Acclimatization doesn't just prepare your limbs. When your mind associates the cold with invigorating activity rather than discomfort, you've primed your mental game. Cold-climate condition isn't solely a physical endeavour; it's where mind and elements meet in a dance of willpower and endurance. A simple start is to take walks in the cold, letting the brisk air nudge your comfort zone wider day by day.

Leverage your workouts through thermogenesis. Engage in high-intensity bursts that ignite your body's furnace. This metabolic trick doesn't just burn calories; it builds a shield against the chill. Your internal engine will keep you warmer longer, and that sustained core heat is key in cold climates. Bodyweight exercises, sprints, or plyometrics are excellent catalysts for this inner fire.

Dress strategically; it's not about the thickest coat but layers you can peel back like the skin of an onion. Start with moisture-wicking materials closest to the skin, insulating layers next, and a breathable, windproof outer shell. Learn the fine art of staying warm without sweating, as dampness can lead to rapid heat loss once you reduce activity intensity.

Hydration is not just for the heat. The air is drier in the winter and dehydration creeps in on silent snowfall. Drink water regularly, your breath fog should remind you—each puff carries away precious moisture. Additionally, ensure your flask can resist freezing.

Fueling for your cold-weather workout requires a tactical approach. Your body burns more fuel to maintain its core temperature, so hearty, energy-rich foods are your best friend. Think complex carbohydrates, healthy fats, and proteins that release energy slowly and keep you fuelled throughout your routine.

Factoring in the shorter days, you'll need to seize the daylight efficiently or become comfortable with the beam of a headlamp. Visibility is key, not just for you but for others who might share the path. And yes, under the cloak of darkness, the cold does bite a touch sharper, making such sessions an even greater test of your determination.

Don't underestimate the value of a proper warm-up indoors before venturing out. Warming up your body can greatly reduce the risk of injury as your muscles will be limber and elastic, not stiff from the cold. Dynamic stretches and light cardio can serve as your prelude to the grand ballet of outdoor fitness.

Embrace activities that are unique to the cold. Snowshoeing, cross-country skiing, even building a snow fort, all require vast energy outlays and reward with a full-body workout. These activities enhance your cold weather resilience by urging you to push against the unique resistance that only a snow-clad landscape can offer.

Clue into the winter's silent language—the whistle of the wind, the firmness of the snow, and how the cold air makes you feel. These signs will guide your routine, telling you when to push harder and when to respect nature's boundaries by easing off. Intuition is a powerful guide when the earth is swathed in white.

Don't shy away from the occasional blizzard—within reason and safety, of course. Training in a gentle snowfall can be enchanting, transforming a regular workout into an otherworldly experience. It's as if the snowflakes cheer you on, each one a whisper of encouragement against the rosy flush of your cheeks.

Post-workout care in the cold differs. You need a swift transition out of damp clothes and into a warm environment. Recovery might entail a warm beverage or a meal that steams with comfort, reinforcing your body's ideal temperature and kick-starting recovery. Sustain your well-being with activities like yoga or gentle stretching that can be done indoors, marrying the frosty outdoor vigour with warmth that nurtures.

Consistency will breed not just success but joy in this frosty regime. The landscape changes daily, clad in diamonds some days, hushed with thick snow on others, offering a panorama of transformative backdrops to your evolving journey. Every cold climate workout can't help but be unique, etching into the memory like patterns of frost upon a windowpane.

As your cold climate conditioning journey unfolds, let it be contagiously inspiring. Share with others the pure elation that comes from a session amongst the flurries. Your breathless tales will stir hearts, encouraging them to lace up their own boots and step into the winter wonderland, where fitness and frost meet in exhilarating harmony.

Chapter 9:
Finding the Right Equipment

As we pivot from mastering the elements to mastering our gear, 'Finding the Right Equipment' becomes a mantra for any enthusiast seeking to fuse nature's unpredictability with the certainty of proper kit. It isn't about splashing out on fancy gadgets; it's about wisely choosing tools that become extensions of our bodies, allies against the whims of Mother Nature. We're not just picking a pair of boots; we're selecting the soles that will tread countless trails. Whether it's finding a breathable waterproof jacket that can shrug off a summer downpour or investing in those resilient gloves that don't stiffen in the frosty breath of winter, every piece of equipment is a silent pledge of our commitment to the great outdoors. It's a delightful ritual—examining, evaluating, and eventually embracing the gear that will carry us through seasons of adventure. As we pore over this chapter's insights into choosing the right gear, remember: be it the whisper of GORE-TEX® or the clink of carabiners, the right equipment is the cornerstone of not just surviving, but thriving in the unique gym nature has bestowed upon us.

Essential Gear for Year-Round Activities

As we journey through the wonders of each season, there's a thrill in knowing you're prepared for anything that nature throws your way. Having the right equipment can make or break your outdoor experience. Let's tuck into the essential gear you'll need, ensuring that you remain comfortable, safe, and free to revel in the great outdoors any day of the year.

First off, a solid pair of footwear is non-negotiable. You'll likely need a few different pairs: lightweight and breathable for those warm, sun-kissed jaunts; waterproof and sturdy for your trots through rain-soaked pathways; and insulated, sure-footed boots for when old man winter casts his chilly spell. Think of your shoes as faithful companions, each one attuned to a season's call.

Your next layer of consideration is clothing. Here, versatility is key. Invest in moisture-wicking fabrics that keep you dry during sweat-inducing summer hikes or unexpected spring downpours. When autumn's crisp air saunters in, layering becomes your strategy for warmth without bulk. And in the depths of winter, thermal and windproof layers are as critical as the fire that warms the hearth. Remember, what you wear directly affects your performance and enjoyment.

Pivotal to your all-season arsenal is the quintessential outer layer: the jacket. It's wise to have a range - a light, windproof shell for blustery days, a waterproof jacket for the deluge, and an insulated coat for temperature plunges. Choosing one with breathable technology will help regulate your body heat, while details like reinforced seams and adjustable hoods can keep the elements firmly outside.

When the sun plays hide and seek, a pair of quality sunglasses will protect your eyes from UV rays, be it glinting off snow or shimmering through trees. Similarly, in low light or after dark, a reliable headlamp or torch can illuminate your path, preventing missteps and guiding the way. Both should be durable and preferably multifunctional, with sunglasses doubling up to shield against wind and a torch that can flash SOS signals if needed.

And where would we be without our trusty backpack? Choose a size that suits your activities – no need for a 50-litre beast on a simple trail run. Look for ones with hydration system compatibility for hands-free sipping, and those with multiple compartments help organise gear effectively. Don't forget comfort – padded straps and a waist belt can distribute weight evenly, saving your back during longer escapades.

Hydration systems themselves can't be overlooked. A water bottle or bladder that's easy to refill, clean, and carry will keep you sipping happily without the hassle. For days out in the heat, consider bottles with insulation to keep your drink cool or, in winter, to prevent it from freezing. Also, a water filtration system might be just what you need for longer, remote trips where the purity of your water source is uncertain.

Your hands deserve some attention too. Gloves, like footwear, call for variety. Lightweight and breathable for hot days, waterproof for rain, and insulated for cold – each pair catering to a tactile connection with nature's ever-changing mood board. Look for touchscreen compatibility in at least one pair so you won't have to bare your hands when it's brisk outside just to use your devices.

Let's talk navigation. A reliable compass or GPS device should always find a place in your pack. You might think you know the trails like the back of your hand, but fog descends, snow covers, and trails vanish. Having the means to orientate yourself in any weather can turn a potential misadventure into a confident stride forward.

And then, there are those extra comfort items – a foldable seat mat or a compact hammock. These can bring a touch of luxury to your rest stops, inviting you to linger longer and soak up the surroundings. They don't take up much space but can add immeasurably to your outdoor experience by offering a warm, dry place to sit or a chance to gently sway among the trees.

For those who revel in their workouts, a weather-resistant fitness tracker is a must. Monitoring your heart rate, the distance covered, and calories burned can stoke that sense of achievement – regardless of weather conditions. Choose a device that syncs with your phone for a seamless integration of technology and nature.

Though often an afterthought, skin protection is vital. Sunscreen is a year-round ally against harmful rays, don't be fooled by overcast days – UV can still reach you. And in the winter, a balm to protect your face from the bite of frosty winds can be a saviour. Pack both, and your future self will thank you when you return from the wilds without a burn or chap in sight.

Lastly, let's not forget the essential tool of recovery – a first aid kit. From minor scratches to more serious cuts, you'll want to be prepared. Make sure it's stocked with antiseptic wipes, plasters, bandages, and any personal medications. It should be compact enough to fit unobtrusively in your pack but accessible enough for a quick response when needed.

There it is – your comprehensive year-round gear guide, each item harmonising to create the perfect outdoor ensemble. Consider it your ticket to a seamless transition through the calendar's pages, experiencing the best of what each season has to offer. So gear up, step out, and let nature's endless playground captivate your heart and invigorate your body – whatever the weather.

Maintaining and Storing Outdoor Equipment

Maintenance is the unsung hero of a long-lasting relationship with your outdoor gear. It's easy to focus on acquiring the latest equipment and pushing ourselves in the adrenaline-rich embrace of the wild. However, the true test of an adventurer's respect for their tools comes in the care they devote after the exhilaration fades. Just as we stretch and rest our weary limbs, our gear too needs tending to ensure it's ready for the next escapade.

Start by establishing a routine to clean equipment post-adventure. All gear, from the humble hiking boot to the more elaborate climbing harness, yearns for a wipe down or a scrub. It may seem tedious, but removing dirt and contaminants can significantly extend the life of your gear. Besides, this ritual allows for a close inspection for wear or damage that could compromise your safety next time you're out there.

Seasonal storage adds another layer to gear longevity. Winter gear, bulky and often with complex structures, requires you to dry everything thoroughly before storing. Moisture is the catalyst for decay and unpleasant odours. Once dried, find a cool, dry place to rest soft goods, and hang things like skis or snowshoes where they're not under stress from straps or weight.

For summer gear, the principle is much the same. Ensure tents are bone-dry before folding for storage to avoid mildew. Sleeping bags should be stored in large, breathable bags, not the compression sacks used for backpacking. This lets insulation maintain loft and warmth. And, just like their winter counterparts, look to hang or properly support equipment that can be deformed or stressed when not in use.

Equipment like ropes, which serve as lifelines in mountainous treks or forays into climbing, demand attentive care. Keep them away from corrosive substances like household chemicals and safeguard from UV radiation by storing them out of sunlight. Also, coiling ropes loosely helps maintain integrity, avoiding kinks and stress points.

Technical gear too has its quirks. Sharpen and oil moving parts when necessary. For your safety devices and tools, double-check their working condition and service them according to the manufacturer's guide. Before storing, remove batteries from electronics to prevent corrosion—and always keep them out of children's reach.

Footwear, often the most abused of all, craves a little TLC. Remove insoles and laces, wash them separately, and let the shoes air out. Consider specialized footwear dryers or stuffing with newspapers to aid the process. High-quality leather boots may also need conditioning, and all types of shoes benefit from a good waterproofing treatment every so often.

Camping stoves and cookware mustn't be overlooked. Clean after every trip, and before long-term storage, ensure they're not only clean but also dry. Fuel should be stored separately, following safety recommendations, and checked for stability over time.

Bikes join the cadre of gear in needing systematic checks and cleaning rituals. Lubrication of the chain, checking tire pressure, and ensuring brake functionality aren't just post-ride tasks but pivotal in off-season storage care. When you tuck your bike away, ensure it doesn't rest solely on the tires, which could lead to warping.

Finally, consider the environment in which you store your beloved gear. A controlled climate is ideal—an area that's neither too dry nor too humid. A consistent temperature extends the life across the board. If pests are a concern, take preventative measures to protect your investment from nibbling critters.

Documentation and tracking can also be a gear geek's best friend. Create a logbook where you record when equipment was purchased, when it was last serviced, and any repairs or upgrades. This meticulous approach not only maintains the gear itself but also your confidence in it.

And while we're talking about confidence, ensure your gear maintains its integrity by not overloading rucksacks, waterproof bags, and other weight-bearing equipment. Respect the weight limits and distribution recommendations to prevent undue stress and potential equipment failure.

Storing gear correctly is a fine balance between accessibility and preservation. You'll want your gear ready to grab when wanderlust strikes, but don't sacrifice its condition for convenience. Plan your storage with the ebb and flow of seasons in mind, rotating gear as needed.

Do not take for granted the peace of mind that comes from well-maintained gear. It sits quietly in the background of every adventure, the silent guardian that keeps mishaps at bay, letting you focus on the beauty of the great outdoors and the richness of experience it offers.

By adopting a diligent approach to maintaining and storing your outdoor equipment, you affirm your commitment not only to the gear itself but to the lifestyle it supports. Look after your tools, and they will repay you with reliability and longevity, becoming trusted companions on many a future journey.

Chapter 10:
Personalising Your Nature's Gym Routine

Stepping into the heart of our discussion, let's pivot to carving out a routine in this alfresco fitness sanctuary that's as unique as your fingerprint. Visualise your existing regime, brimming with reps and sets, then scatter it amongst the trees, letting the land's contours shape your exertions. Crafting this personal tapestry weaves together your well-being with the undulating pulse of the earth. It isn't about lifting the heaviest stones; it's about listening to your rhythm and mirroring the natural flux around you. Whether you're scaling a rugged trail or pacing by the river's edge, attune your workouts to your deepest inclinations—let your heartbeat synchronise with the rustle of leaves and your breath echo the whispers of the wind. With each session, your narrative unfolds, creating a symphony of movement that celebrates the vitality of both your spirit and the living, breathing gym around you. Here, in the wild's embrace, your fitness odyssey becomes a personal revolution, flowering with every sunrise you chase and every horizon you greet.

Assessing Fitness Levels and Goals

As we lace up our boots or set our sights on the looming mountain trail, it's essential to turn an inward gaze to our current fitness levels and the ambitions that fuel our strides. Embarking on the journey of outdoor activities isn't just about responding to the call of the wild; it's inherently tied to personal challenges and milestones we aim to achieve. Hence, it's paramount to assess where we stand and chart our course with a compass of clarity.

Firstly, gauging fitness levels can be an exploratory exercise in itself. Whether you can take on a steep incline without losing your breath or if a leisurely hike is more your pace, it's all about starting from a realistic perspective. Let's not be overly critical, yet it's crucial to avoid donning rose-tinted glasses when it comes to our physical capabilities.

A sensible approach is to consider previous experiences. Have you found yourself gasping for air after a short jog or do you comfortably conquer kilometres with breath to spare? Also, ponder on how often you currently engage in any physical activity. Consistency can be a more reliable indicator of fitness than sporadic bursts of exertion.

It doesn't take sophisticated equipment to perform a basic assessment—simple exercises like push-ups, squats, or a timed walk can provide a wealth of information about your stamina, strength, and endurance. If these seem daunting, ease in with activities more aligned with your comfort level, such as brisk walks or gentle yoga sequences.

Understanding your body's boundaries would be incomplete without factoring in flexibility and balance—critical components for outdoor escapades. Stretch regularly and test yourself with one-legged stands or dynamic movements to see how swiftly and gracefully you can navigate uneven terrains.

Next, let's dive into goals. Goals, like the North Star, should guide our engagements with the great outdoors. They can be as varied as the landscapes we yearn to explore—from mastering a particular trail to enhancing general well-being or dropping a clothes size. Whatever the endgame, setting SMART goals (Specific, Measurable, Achievable, Relevant, Time-bound) can transform nebulous dreams into palpable targets.

But remember, the beauty of outdoor activities is that they need not be confined to mere physical achievements. Deepening your connection with nature or finding mental serenity under the canopy of ancient trees can be as significant as any number on a scale or stopwatch.

While we're on the subject, let's mull over milestones and markers of progress. It's rejuvenating to celebrate the gradual increases in distance trekked or the enhanced ease at which you now ascend slopes. Just like the changing of seasons, progress might ebb and flow; the key is to relish both the dramatic leaps and the subtle shifts.

Moreover, flexibility in goals is imperative. Perhaps you initially desired to summit peaks but find yourself enamoured by the poetic rhythm of long-distance running through feathered meadows. It's okay for passions to evolve, and with them, your goals. Outdoor fitness is less about rigidity and more about the fluid dance with nature's ever-shifting panoramas.

Retaining a log or a journal can be instrumental in this adventure. Not only does it put into perspective the ground covered, but it also stands testament to your growing bond with the wilderness. Jot down thoughts, tally hikes, or sketch the curve of the hills you've crested— the choice is yours, as personal as the journey.

Annual reflection is another gem worth incorporating into this process. Just like trees shed their leaves and bloom anew, taking stock yearly helps to appreciate growth and refresh or revise goals. This could coincide with the New Year or any significant date that prompts you to pause and ponder.

In seeking guidance or structuring your approach, there's no shame in reaching out. A like-minded community or a seasoned guide can shed light on blind spots and foster a supportive environment to thrive in. After all, every great explorer once had a map drawn up by someone who tread the path before them.

Don't let setbacks unravel you either. Twists, turns, and the occasional stumble are as much a part of the journey as the victories. They're not a sign to retreat but to stand up, dust yourself off, and find a pace that better suits the present moment.

In conclusion, stepping into nature's gym requires that we not only map the external but also navigate the contours of our own aspirations and physicality. It's a balance of respecting where we are while reaching earnestly for the peaks we wish to conquer. As you etch your path, remember, the mountains, forests, and rivers are patient; they've stood for eons and will bear witness to your story of progress, perseverance, and the pursuit of wellness, wrapped in the embrace of the Earth's splendour.

With fitness levels assessed and goals set, we are ready to delve into the integration of our passions and hobbies with our newfound fitness regimen. But that is a tale for another time, for another chapter in this adventure that we write with every step into the wild.

Combining Passions: Integrating Hobbies with Fitness

For those of you seeking to merge your leisurely pursuits with a fitness agenda, integrating hobbies with fitness isn't just a pie-in-the-sky idea; it's a tangible, enriching path to a healthier lifestyle. Consider for a moment the simple joy of a hobby. Doesn't matter if it's bird watching, photography, gardening, or stargazing - these are passions that light up the soul. Now imagine adding a layer of physical activity to these interests. That's where the magic happens.

The secret behind fusing hobbies with fitness is to look for the natural synergy between physical movement and your favourite pastimes. Let's take photography as an example. Gone are the days when photography is just about light and composition; it can also be about treks through the countryside, scaling hills or waiting patiently in nature – all fantastic forms of exercise that engage different muscle groups and challenge your endurance.

Or perhaps your idea of a perfect day includes some time spent with flora. Gardening, often overlooked as a hobby with fitness benefits, is actually a fantastic way to get a full-body workout. Digging, planting, weeding, and cutting are all actions that utilise the major muscle groups, and doing them consistently can certainly count as a workout. The trick is to approach your garden session with an awareness of the physical effort involved, turning each movement into a conscious exercise.

Those with a love of the cosmos might spend nights gazing at the stars. Sounds sedentary? Not necessarily. Consider cycling to a remote star-gazing spot or walking a hiking trail before settling down to watch the night sky. Suddenly, a tranquil hobby takes on a new dimension of activity, boosting your heart rate before quieting your mind with the infinity above.

Avid readers can even turn their love for books into a fitness challenge. Audio books or podcasts allow the flexibility to absorb the written word while on the move. Why not listen to the next chapter of a gripping novel while jogging through the park, or learning from a motivational podcast on a brisk walk? It's an excellent way to keep both mind and body engaged.

For the musically inclined, dancing is an obvious choice; yet, there are other ways to combine music with movement. Drummers or percussion enthusiasts could explore drumming circles where they can play while moving around the circle, incorporating dance and rhythm into the exercise session, while wind and brass players could practice their breath control while engaging in light cardiovascular activities like walking.

Culinary buffs might enjoy the fitness aspect of foraging for their ingredients. It's not only an intensive scavenger hunt across different terrains but also a brilliant way to understand the source of your food. The act of foraging can be both physically demanding and mentally stimulating, as you require knowledge of the land and the seasonality of its produce.

For those who weave magic with thread and yarn, have you considered taking your knitting or crocheting outdoors? Holding sitting positions during these activities strengthens the core, and doing them perched on a rock or log in the middle of a forest adds a balance challenge to the task. Plus, the dose of fresh air does wonders for creativity!

Animal lovers can combine their affection for four-legged friends with staying active. Horseback riding, running with your dog, or simply setting off on a wildlife-seeking hike can satisfy both your need for company and exercise. It's about creative thinking - ponder for a moment how your love for animals can lead to a physically active lifestyle.

Even video game aficionados can get in on the action. While traditional gaming is a sedentary hobby, there's a burgeoning world of movement-based games that require full-body interaction. Geocaching, a real-world, outdoor treasure hunting game using GPS-enabled devices, offers a perfect blend of tech and exercise. Alternatively, create a workout challenge for every level you beat or set a timer to jog in place between game sessions.

Bird watchers, too, can attest to the incidental fitness walking through wetlands, forests, and fields in pursuit of elusive feathered creatures. It's not just about the stillness in waiting but the journey to the watch point that gets the heart going. You see, the idea isn't to revamp your hobby into a workout. It's about enhancing it with an active component that feels as natural as the hobby itself.

Sailing enthusiasts are blessed with a hobby that's inherently physical. The hauling of ropes and the balancing necessitated by the ebb and flow of the waves contribute to a significant workout. It illustrates how some hobbies already come with a fitness bonus - the key is to be aware of it and maybe push a little harder next time you're out on the water.

What we're suggesting here isn't about crossing the finish line fastest or lifting the heaviest weights. We're talking about celebrating movement and integrating it with what you already love doing. It's cultivating a dual passion where your hobby enriches your fitness routine, and your fitness adds depth to your hobby.

By considering how you can integrate your hobby with added physicality, you start down a road that makes fitness an intrinsic part of who you are. It's a lifestyle choice that makes your heart as happy as it is healthy. Layer in the twists and turns of the seasons, and suddenly, you have a dynamic, year-round program that flawlessly blends your interests with overall well-being.

So, whether you're aiming to merge tranquil pursuits or are looking to rev up your adrenaline-packed activities, remember that your hobbies shouldn't be seen as separate from your fitness journey. They can work hand in hand, carving out a wonderfully holistic approach to staying active and satisfied across all seasons. Go ahead, get creative, and let the lines between fitness and fun blissfully blur!

Chapter 11:
Staying Motivated Through the Seasons

Staying motivated as the months roll by isn't just about gritting your teeth and pushing through. It's about tuning into the *rhythms of nature*, finding your flow amidst the ebb and flow of seasons. Whether you're basking in the golden glow of summer or wrapping up against the crisp whisper of winter chill, there's a secret recipe for keeping your spirit high and your body in motion. Harness each season's unique offerings; **let the bursting life of spring** feed into your strides, **let autumn's tapestry of colours** enliven your workout backdrop, and find solace in **winter's serene whites** for reflection and building inner strength. Understanding that variety is the spice of life, our motivation must be seasoned with variety too. Through the rain's gentle rhythm or the snow's muffled hush, we continue—not because we must, but because we are moved by the *ever-changing canvas* that invites us to be part of it.

Setting and Tracking Seasonal Objectives

As we transition from one chapter to the next, just as we do from season to season, it's essential to reflect on our progress and chart a course for the future. So imagine the fresh possibilities each season brings, a constant cycle of renewal that beckons you to set new benchmarks for your outdoor journey.

But how does one capture the essence of each season, with its unique challenges and opportunities, and distil it into meaningful goals? It's not just about plucking an aim from the frosty winter air or the warm spring breeze; it's about crafting objectives that resonate with the rhythm of the seasons and your own personal growth.

Let's start with spring, the time of new beginnings. Here lies the perfect chance to awaken dormant aspirations. The soft crunch of boots on a dewy morning trail—consider this your cue to step up your distance or try a new outdoor activity. As flowers unfurl, let's aim to stretch our capabilities, setting goals that push our limits, yet are as attainable as the next bloom.

As summer's fiery embrace takes hold, our objectives might shift towards endurance, making the most of extended daylight to explore further, longer, deeper. At this time, tracking your achievements can be as simple as noting the extra mile you jogged on the beach or the new swimming stroke you've mastered in the cool embrace of a lake.

Autumn whispers a tale of transformation, and with it, our goals should adapt. Perhaps it's time to transition to more meditative exercises, such as tai chi beneath the burnished canopy of a forest. Tracking progress in fall might mean reflecting on how these practices improve mental clarity and prepare you for the inward focus winter often demands.

Winter, with its crisp clarity, invites us to fortify our inner resilience. Can you outpace your previous cold-weather workouts, or find the courage to try ice-climbing? Your tracking could be a brave diary of venturing out, despite the inviting warmth of the indoors. Evaluate not just physical achievement, but also the mental toughness you're cultivating.

To effectively chart our seasonal goals and track them, the first step is clear articulation. Be specific. "Improve stamina" is a noble aspiration, but "Increase my regular hike by 2 kilometres by the end of spring" gives you a tangible target and timeline. Write it down, pin it up – make it real. Make it visible.

Then, measure meticulously. Whether you choose a classic journal, an app, or a giant calendar on the wall, select a method that inspires consistency in your documentation. Regularly jotting down the weather conditions, your emotions, the vividness of your surroundings—all of this enhances the narrative of your journey and the progress towards your goals.

Consider the tools you'll use. From pedometers and fitness trackers that count steps and monitor heart rates to more advanced GPS devices that map out your trails, technology can be your ally in pursuit of your seasonal aspirations. But don't let it overshadow the importance of intuition and mindfulness in gauging your achievements.

Accountability partners or groups can be instrumental in keeping your sights set on your objectives. Find a friend whose goals align with yours, or join a community of outdoor enthusiasts who share updates and encouragement. The collective spirit of achieving goals can often propel you past points where you might falter alone.

It's also about adaptability. Be willing to revise your goals as the seasons and your circumstances shift. If summer blazes too fiercely for that midday run, shift your strategy—seek the cool of dawn or dusk. It's not conceding defeat; it's intelligently adjusting to the ebb and flow of natural cycles.

And let's not forget to celebrate the milestones, no matter how modest. An extra lap around the park, a steeper climb conquered, these triumphs are the incremental victories that bring us closer to our larger vision. Every celebrated success fuels your motivation for the next season's objectives.

When setting your sights on a new goal, imagine how it will feel to reach it amidst the changing backdrop of the seasons. Visualise the satisfaction of achieving a new personal best in the balmy embrace of a summer's evening or the peace of a yoga pose held steady amid the rustling whispers of autumn leaves.

Above all, remember that these objectives aren't just etchings on the year's calendar—they're signposts of your evolving relationship with nature and yourself. The numbers, the achieved distances, the conquered fears all tell a story that is uniquely yours.

So as one season dovetails into the next, peer into your well of objectives. Extract from it a goal that harmonises with the season's symphony and your life's melody. And when you've soared past your target, take solace in the fact that soon enough the cycle recommences—a fresh canvas of snow, a burst of spring greenery, a golden autumnal leaf carpet, or a pristine summer dawn—to nurture the seeds of new dreams.

In the end, setting and tracking seasonal objectives isn't just about fitness or outdoor activity—it's a celebration of the passage of time and personal growth. It's a journey taken on the ever-changing terrain of life, where each new objective paves the way for seasons of discovery, resilience, joy, and serenity.

Overcoming Seasonal Affective Barriers

When the days shorten and temperatures plummet, it's common to feel the winter blues, isn't it? Seasonal affective disorder (SAD) isn't just an excuse; it's a clinically recognised condition that can substantially impede our motivation to stay fit and connect with the great outdoors. Yet, here lies our opportunity to break from the confines of gloomy moods and claim back the rejuvenating power of nature—regardless of snowflakes or chilling winds.

Firstly, recognizing the signs of SAD is vital for tackling its effects head-on. It may express itself as a persistent low mood, a loss of pleasure in everyday activities, or a general feeling of lethargy. You might even find yourself withdrawing from your once-loved nature excursions. Noticing these changes is the crucial first step in creating a battle plan that keeps your outdoor pursuits in constant motion.

One of the most effective strategies involves maximizing exposure to natural light. Even on the shortest days, a brief lunchtime walk can work wonders. It's imperative to align your schedule with the daylight hours, sneaking in those moments of sunshine whenever the opportunity arises. Despite the chill, just a short sojourn outside can uplift mood and sharpen mental focus.

Nutrition plays a powerful supporting role in overcoming the barriers set by SAD. Foods rich in omega-3 fatty acids, vitamin D, and B vitamins can help boost mood and energy levels. Tailoring your diet to include these nutrients may give you the extra edge you need to lace up those boots and step out the door, even when the comfort of home tempts you to stay put.

Exercise, without a doubt, is a stalwart ally in the fight against seasonal depression. However, the connection between physical activity and improved mood is magnified when exercise is performed outdoors. Whether it's a steady jog on a frosty morning or a vigorous snowshoe hike, the endorphin release combined with the sensory experience of the natural environment can be a potent mood-lifter.

Sometimes, a change in perspective is all that's needed to break through the mental barriers. Winter's landscape presents a unique canvas—one that's only available for a fraction of the year. Embrace the rarity of frozen lakes, the tranquillity of snow-dusted forests, and the quietness that comes when much of the wildlife is hibernating. It's a chance to see your familiar trails afresh.

Setting incremental, achievable targets can also help maintain outdoor exercise habits. Aiming to cover a certain number of miles every week or exploring a new trail can provide a compelling reason to brave the chill. Tracking these small victories not only instils a sense of accomplishment but also a tangible record of your persistence against seasonal challenges.

Finding camaraderie in group activities may be the encouragement needed to persist through winter woes. Organising a weekly group hike or joining a community running club provides both social interaction and accountability. The shared experience of enduring brisk conditions can fortify friendships and fortify your resolve to stay active.

Layering appropriately doesn't only apply to clothing. It's also about layering your activities; begin with a brisk walk, add some light jogging intervals, and maybe integrate body-weight exercises at scenic points. This variety keeps things interesting and your body warm, effectively turning nature's chill into an ally for fitness.

Never underestimate the power of visualization and mindfulness as tools to conquer seasonal barriers. A visualization practice where you imagine the sights, sounds, and sensations of a lush spring jog can prime your motivation on drab winter mornings. Likewise, mindfulness exercises rooted in acceptance and the embracing of seasonal changes can reset your mental compass towards positivity and action.

Remember, the challenge of cold weather is temporary. Spring is always waiting on the other side, promising longer days and warmer climates. Sustaining outdoor activities through the winter prepares you physically and mentally to leap into spring with vitality and enthusiasm. You'll be primed to hit the ground running, often literally, as the thaw arrives.

For those days when the weather becomes especially prohibitive, keeping a routine flexible is key. It could mean opting for an indoor workout that simulates the outdoor experience. Perhaps a yoga session with a visual backdrop of a serene forest, or a treadmill run set to the sounds of chirping birds. This keeps the connection with nature's rhythms alive in your heart and mind.

Don't shy away from seeking professional support if SAD grips tightly. It's not a sign of weakness but one of self-care and determination. Sometimes a conversation with a health professional can bring clarity and additional coping strategies that enable us to thrive during all seasons.

Above all, it's essential to maintain a gentle spirit of patience with oneself. Some days might feel like a step backwards; it's all part of the dance with nature. Acknowledge the feeling, wrap up warmly, and consider each outdoor venture as an act of triumph over the seasonal affective barriers.

Embracing the cold months as an opportunity rather than a hurdle can fundamentally shift your experiences with nature. Winter offers a distinctive beauty and quiet, allowing for profound interaction with the world around you. It's a season that bestows a unique strength and resilience, both in our environment and within ourselves.

Ultimately, it's about harnessing the same tenacity that nature demonstrates as it endures and adapts to winter. Just as the resilient pine stands strong against the snow, so too can we. Overcoming seasonal affective barriers is not just about enduring winter; it's about thriving within it, finding joy in the crunch of snow beneath our boots, and the crisp air that fills our lungs. It's another beautiful chapter in our ongoing story of well-being through nature's gym.

Nature's Playlists: Musical Motivation for All Weathers

Now let's delve into the power of music to fuel our workouts and harmonise with the varying moods of Mother Nature. It might sound a bit fantastical, but think about it: have you ever found your stride hit a perfect tempo with a great tune during a run, or felt your spirits lift while cycling to a pounding beat?

Indeed, music can be a transformative force, animating our outdoor pursuits whether the skies are blue or grey. It's the pulse to our proverbial dance with the elements—an untapped resource for all who seek a deepened connection with both themselves and the weather-beaten paths.

Imagine a drizzly spring morning—the kind that whispers of renewal but suggests you'd be better off under the covers. Yet, armed with a playlist that boasts the vibrant melodies of birdsong set to an up-tempo harmony, you're inspired to lace up and become part of the awakening landscape.

In the heat of the summer, when the sun's rays play with the shade, your tracks mirror this interplay of light and heat. Calypso rhythms or sultry jazz can accompany your beach runs, infusing your steps with the nonchalance of a sun-drenched afternoon, making the heat feel like a welcome embrace rather than an adversary.

Autumn brings a different tune: the rustle of leaves and the crispness in the air. Your playlist then could be a reflection of change and introspection—a rhythmic yet comforting collection of acoustics that urge you to keep moving through the hues of change.

Winter, with its stark beauty, often dares us to brave the chill. Here's where the warm tones of an instrumental crescendo can be your ally against the cold, their reverberating baseline matching the crunch of snow underfoot as you make your way through a frosty world, seemingly asleep.

In contrast, when faced with rain and mists, it's the deeper sounds—a mix of synth and calm, fluid beats—that can transform a soggy landscape into a mystic adventure. They're the perfect companion to the tap-tap-tapping of raindrops on your waterproofs as you jog through the liquid world.

With the wind comes its own soundtrack, a symphony capable of embodying its fickle gusts. An eclectic mix with crescendos matching the wind's playful pushes can help you embrace the challenge and use the resistance as a novel motivator.

When winter resurfaces with ice and snow, the sounds from your speakers should be as crisp as the air your breath forms in – stark and pure. Here, a classical piece can parallel the tranquil solitude of a snow-covered vista, whilst an electronic beat matches the crackle of ice beneath your boots.

But it's not just about slapping together a few favourite tracks. Crafting a playlist is an art, a personal curation that aligns with your heartbeat, your breath, and the cadence of your footfalls. It's a blend of science and soul, tempo and emotion, designed to propel you through any season's offering.

Envisage a tempo that's in sync with the pitter-patter of rain or the howl of the wind. Songs that can adjust your stride just enough to turn the battle with the breeze into a dance. Tunes that echo the squelch of mud underfoot, endorsing the earthy reality of nature's softer, wetter days.

And for those snow-laden landscapes? Don't underestimate the power of a robust rock anthem or the defiance of an electrifying guitar solos. They can make the biting cold feel like a mere backdrop to an epic chapter in your fitness journey.

Let's not forget the psychological dimension of this musical adventure. It's not just the physical push but the mental shove that's often needed. The right songs can whisper encouragement when the skies growl or offer solace when isolation weighs heavy on a solo trek.

The trick is in knowing that the tempo of your tunes should mirror, or even dictate, the pace of your workout. A study or two have shown that we're slaves to rhythm—and stepping in time with music can not only improve your exercise efficiency but also make the endeavour more enjoyable. And isn't that, after all, the golden ticket?

Where to begin, then, with this symphony of steps and seasons? Start simple—a song for the warm-up that feels like the first rays of sunlight through leaves, a high-energy track for the peak of your exertion that rivals even the mightiest of storms, and a mellow melody for cool-down that's akin to the gentle pattering of the first fall of snow.

So let the skies set the cue. Next time you're faced with a dalliance outdoors, pause. What's the weather telling you, and what tunes can be the overture to your day's journey? As the cycle of seasons spins, your nature's playlist becomes your steadfast motivator, your melodic coach, and most importantly, your companion through every drop of rain, every ray of sun, every gust of wind, and every flake of snow.

Chapter 12:
Nutrition for the Seasons

As we turn over the leaf to a fresh page, let's delve into the transformative power of eating in harmony with the calendar's ebb and flow. In **"Nutrition for the Seasons"**, we explore how the changing environment intricately weaves into the tapestry of what fuels our bodies. Each season parades its own bounty—not merely a feast for the eyes but a cornucopia of nutrients catering to our body's evolving needs as we tackle the elements head-on. Whether it's the verdant greens rejuvenating us through spring, the vibrant berries fuelling our summer adventures, or the roots and squashes storing energy for our autumn hikes, each offers its unique whispers of wisdom. And let's not forget the hearty connections in winter—where slow-cooked stews remind us of the Earth's slumber beneath the frost. Hydration, too, shifts with the mercury; from sipping cool, mint-infused water under the scorching sun to cradling a steaming mug after braving a snow-laden trail—it's not just about quenching thirst, it's about nourishing every cell to revel in the great outdoors. Wrapping ourselves in nature's rhythmic diet, we tap into an ancient source of vitality, sharpening our endurance against the clarion call of the wilderness.

Eating Seasonally: Fuel for Outdoor Workouts

As we continue to journey through the exploration of nature's gym and the vibrant transition from one season to the next, let's delve into the role of seasonal eating. Making intentional food choices in alignment with the seasons is not just beneficial for our planet—it's optimal for fuelling our bodies when we engage in outdoor workouts.

Eating with the seasons allows us to consume produce when it's at its prime. This means fresher, more nutritious, and often tastier ingredients that work in harmony with our body's seasonal needs. In summer, for example, our bodies often crave light, water-rich fruits and vegetables to stay hydrated and cool. Winter calls for denser, calorie-rich foods to provide the extra energy needed to battle the cold.

Picture this: you've planned a long hike on a crisp autumn morning. Wouldn't it feel instinctively right to start your day with a hearty breakfast of porridge topped with cinnamon-spiced apples? Autumn's harvest gifts us with squashes, roots, and fruits, each packed with vitamins and slow-releasing carbohydrates that are not just delicious but also an ideal base for sustained energy release.

When the blossoms of spring are in full bloom, the earth sprouts new life and the markets teem with the likes of tender greens and berries. A vibrant salad packed with leafy greens, spiced nuts, and a variety of these fresh berries is not only visually inviting but also offers a wealth of antioxidants and nutrients to keep your muscles functioning optimally.

Let's not forget the cooling and hydrating foods of summer. Engaging in vigorous activities like cycling or beach volleyball under the blazing sun demands hydration above all. Integrating watermelon slices, cucumber, and berries into your summer diet can provide a refreshing and replenishing boost. The high water content in these choices helps to replace the fluids lost through sweat, keeping you energised and preventing dehydration.

In the heart of winter, with its short days and relentless chill, your body expends more energy to stay warm. Here, nutrient-dense stews and casseroles can be your best friend. Combine seasonal root vegetables such as parsnips, turnips and sweet potatoes with beans or meat in a slow cooker before you head out for a snowy trail run. You'll return to a warm and fulfilling meal that replenishes the high-calorie deficit and soothes the soul.

The idea of eating seasonally also fosters a unique connection with nature and the cycle of life. As you consume the fruits of the season, there's a certain rhythm that begins to take shape in your dietary habits, mirroring the ebbs and flows of your outdoor activities.

Moreover, seasonal eating does not have to be a mundane task. It's a creative challenge. Think of whipping up a berry and chia seed smoothie after a brisk summer swim, or sipping on a pumpkin-spiced latte post a chilly fall mountain bike ride. The variety offered by seasonal produce means your palate never gets bored, and your body gets a diverse range of nutrients year-round.

It's important to note, however, that eating seasonally doesn't mean restricting yourself unreasonably. The modern world offers choice and variety, but complementing these with local and seasonal produce where possible can help to minimise your ecological footprint and support local economies.

One also has to consider that seasonal eating can require some flexibility and creativity, especially if your local climate is less varied or if certain produce is not readily available. However, the core principle remains: Choose fresh, choose local, and listen to what your body needs in step with the outdoor tasks you undertake.

When we talk about eating seasonally for outdoor workouts, we also need to touch on the pre- and post-exercise foods. Before you set off, a meal balanced in carbohydrates and proteins can give you the right kind of fuel. Post-workout, opt for something rich in protein and fibre to aid recovery. And with each of these meals, let the season be your guide.

Consider the practicality too—outdoor workouts can occasionally be extended affairs. So, packing snacks like nuts and seeds or homemade fruit and oat bars, depending on the time of year, can provide that much-needed energy top-up and keep you going until it's time for a full meal.

If this has sparked a curiosity in you, why not start experimenting with this season's harvest? You could toss a new vegetable into your next stir-fry or snack on some seasonal fruit before heading out for your run. Let the colourful spectrum of nature's produce fuel both your body and your spirit as you work out under the grand, open sky.

In conclusion, making an effort to eat seasonally aligns our physical needs with the natural world's offerings. It's a holistic way to look at fueling our workouts and our lives. Whether you're paddling against the spring tide, scaling sun-soaked cliffs, crunching through autumn leaves or braving the snowy silence of winter trails—the right seasonal food can transform your outdoor experience, adding a deep sense of satisfaction and wellness to your adventures.

Hydration Across Climates: From Humid to Dry

As we wander and work our way through changing scenery, the rhythm of our steps syncs with the beat of nature's heart, yet our bodies' needs for hydration remain a constant amidst this beautiful flux. Now, let's delve into the essential fluidity of life across various climates, from the sultry breathe-easy warmth of humid landscapes to the crisp embrace of arid regions.

Take the humid tropics, where moisture hangs in the air like a blanket. Every movement feels resistant, every pore on your skin breathes out and fails to breathe in fully. While you may not feel thirsty as often due to the ubiquitous moisture, your body loses water rapidly through sweat that doesn't evaporate as easily. It becomes critical to sip water regularly, even if you're not feeling parched, keeping in mind to replace not just the water but also the electrolytes your body expends laboriously.

Conversely, stepping into dry climates can be a deceptive experience. The air, thirsty itself, drinks up your sweat almost as quickly as it appears. This covert loss of fluids doesn't drench you as the tropics do, yet, paradoxically, it's here in the deceptive dryness that dehydration likes to sneak up on you. You must be proactive, drinking water at intervals, because once you feel thirst scratching your throat, dehydration has already begun its wily dance.

It's not just about the volume of water though, it's the how and the when that also counts. Starting your hike or run hydrated sets the stage. Pre-hydrating, the act of drinking fluids before exposure to the elements, makes a noticeable difference. Imagine your body a sponge; pre-soaking it ensures that it's capable of holding more water for a longer period, delaying the effects of dehydration.

Now, you might ponder the merit of plain water against the vast array of sports drinks. It's quite simple, for shorter, less intense exercises, water does the trick. But when you're embarking on longer bouts of exertion or sweating profusely, it's wise to consider concoctions that boast electrolytes – these are akin to your body's spark plugs and are crucial for muscle function.

On the subject of hydration, let's not forget about the little ones. Kids, often swept up in the exhilaration of play, can easily neglect to drink. Subtly guiding them to take sips and offering refreshing fruits like watermelon or orange slices can serve as both a snack and a stealthy hydration tactic. Remember, kids tend to be more vulnerable to temperature extremes, which makes keen observation of their hydration habits all the more vital.

For the endurance enthusiasts who thrive on pushing boundaries, water carriers become as much a part of the gear as their footwear. Be it a hydration backpack or a running belt with bottles, the idea is to make accessing fluids seamless. It's not just about convenience; it's critical strategy – it's the acknowledgement that water is your enduring companion, come hill or high sun.

Moving on from water, we must also tip our hats to the protective role of clothing. Clothing that promotes evaporation, that 'breathes,' essentially assists in our internal cooling process. In humid conditions, look for moisture-wicking fabrics that draw sweat away from the skin and in dry climates, employ light-coloured and loose-fitting garb to reflect the sun's fury away from you. However, don't be fooled – sun-protective clothing doesn't mean you can skimp on water. They're partners in crime, your dual guardians against the heat.

For every morning you wake to an eager sun or a subtle breeze, consider the air's humidity or lack thereof and plan your hydration accordingly. Perhaps today, you'll freeze a bottle of water to take along for your scorching desert trek — the ice slowly melting to match your need for cool sips — or perhaps you'll pack an extra flask to counteract the dense, wet air of the rainforest.

Your dietary intake prior to exposure is another silent player in your hydration game. Consuming foods high in water content can aid your hydration levels before you even take your first step outdoors. Think of cucumbers, strawberries, and peaches not just as tantalizing treats but as aqua-packed partners that aid your quest for balance.

We've explored climates and hydration, but altitude can't be ignored — the higher you ascend, the harder your body works, and the more it craves moisture. Ascending that mountain pass or those high trails necessitates a closer alliance with your water bottle. Don't underestimate the power of elevation; respect it with a steady dribble of water intake as you climb higher into the heavens.

Now let's not overlook the simple pleasure of a cup of tea or a juicy piece of fruit during a rest break. While these moments nourish the soul, they also surreptitiously contribute to your fluid intake. Even sipping on a warm herbal brew at altitude can assist in keeping the body's hydration in check, especially in colder environments where thirst response is often dulled.

Reflection, naturally, leads us back to our roots, to the simplest of truths. Water is life; our very cells dance in it, thrive in it. Out here, amidst the serene or the wild, we must listen to our bodies' quiet cues, sip by sip, beat by beat. Feel the pulse of the land underfoot and the rhythm of your body in unison, harmoniously hydrated, whether in a mist-kissed jungle or beneath the vast desert sky.

And when the sun sets, regardless of the panorama, you'll be glad for the diligence you paid to hydration. The setting sun's colours seem more vibrant, and the cool evening air hits differently when your body is fluid and your mind untroubled by the worry of dehydration. Those final steps of the day's journey are savoured, just as each drop of water was throughout your adventure.

Let's not just move through landscapes; let's understand them, feel them, and respect the role of water every step of the way. Embracing hydration strategies tailored to different climates is to pledge allegiance to both your health and your truest nature—making every inhale an exploration and every exhale a grateful homage to the journey that is life.

Chapter 13:
The Solitary Explorer

Venturing into the wild alone can be as daunting as it is mesmerising; it's here, in the embrace of nature's vastness, where you'll find a unique brand of self-discovery. Picture this: it's just you, the rhythmic cadence of your footsteps, and the undisturbed serenity that cloaks you like an invisible mantle. Solo workouts gift you a precious psychology of alone time that's essential for introspection – and let's face it, there's a particular triumph that courses through your veins when you navigate a trail or conquer a hill without a cheer squad. But let's not wander off the path of caution; being a lone adventurer is heady with freedom, yet it comes with the solemn responsibility to keep safety at your forefront. It's about being prepared – both in mind and gear – for what Mother Nature might whimsically throw your way, be it a sudden change in weather or an unexpected encounter with her wilder inhabitants. Embracing solitude amidst the great outdoors isn't running from the world; it's running deeper into the essence of what it means to be truly alive, attuned not just to your surroundings, but to the deeper rhythms of your own existence.

Solo Workouts: The Psychology of Alone Time in Nature

Venturing into the outdoors alone may seem a daunting prospect to some, yet it reveals itself as a sanctuary of self-discovery and mental reinforcement for those who embrace the solitary path. The beauty found in solo workouts in nature lies not only in the physical exertion but also in the mental fortitude one develops amidst the whispers of the wind and rustling of leaves. This chapter voyages into the depths of that experience, illuminating the psychological aspects of finding one's rhythm in the gentle chaos of nature's own gymnasium.

There's a special kind of dialogue that occurs when you're alone in the vast expanse of nature. Each breath you take speaks to the trees, and with every footfall on the earthen track, you're stitching your story into the fabric of the landscape. Solo workouts invite a meditative state, where the mind can wander, contemplate life's intricacies, or simply exist in the moment, uncluttered by the noise of societal demands or the cadence of conversation. It's in these moments of solitude that many find clarity.

Even more fascinating is the way solo exertion mirrors the larger journey through life itself. There's something raw and authentic about mustering the will to push through physical barriers when you've only got your inner voice as a coach. The external rewards may be absent, no cheers or medals bestowed, but what you receive in return is an intimate understanding of your own strengths and limitations.

For some, the thought of loneliness comes barreling in with the mention of 'alone time'. However, distinguishing between loneliness and solitude is essential here. Loneliness can feel like an unwelcome isolation, a hollow companion; whereas solitude in nature is the nourishing quiet, the mindful pause in life's busy script. It's in these pockets of solitude where personal growth sprouts and flourishes, unencumbered.

It's also about resilience. When the trails get tough and the weather turns, you're your own savior. There's a profound sense of accomplishment when you've weathered the storm solo, proving to yourself that you've got what it takes to overcome even when there's no one to lean on but yourself. This resilience built in solitude often seeps into other areas of life, bolstering confidence and self-reliance.

Let's not sidestep the reality that solo workouts can also foster a deepened sense of awareness. Being singular in the outdoors not only heightens your senses but also compels you to fully understand your surroundings. You're more likely to notice the small wonders: the dew on a spider's web, the shifting patterns of clouds, the way the sunlight dapples through the treetops. This acute awareness can transform into a heightened appreciation for the world around you, potentially stirring a more profound environmental consciousness.

There is, of course, a rhythmic beauty in the solitude of nature's vast gym. Each solo workout is a dance with the elements, a step-to-step match with the uneven terrain. It's not only about conquering landscapes but also about moving in harmony with them, learning the subtle cues that the environment shares. Appreciating this can lead to a more immersive and interactive workout experience.

Emotionally, alone time in nature can act as a reset button. It's a practice that affords the space to process emotions, to run alongside your thoughts rather than from them. The cathartic effect of exerting the body while liberating the mind from everyday stressors is a therapeutic recipe, one that nourishes the soul and cleanses the psyche.

Motivation often becomes more intrinsic when you're by yourself in nature. With no one else to set the pace or dictate the agenda, you're sculpting your own journey, step by step. This self-propelled motivation can forge a robust sense of personal accountability and discipline that's essential in any fitness journey or life endeavor.

Critical too is the aspect of safety, a point we'll explore in greater depth elsewhere. But for now, understand that solo workouts demand smart planning and self-reliance. There's a certain pride in knowing you've equipped yourself to handle what mother nature may hurl your way. The confidence gained from this preparation can be life-affirming.

In the same vein, solo workouts often lead to a better understanding of one's body. The quiet allows for tuning into one's physical state more deeply, recognizing the signs of fatigue or injury quickly, and more importantly, understanding when to push limits and when to reel back. This intimate body awareness is one of the cornerstones of a successful solitary workout regime.

Adventure and the thrill of exploration can't be overlooked as part of the psychology behind solo workouts. Whether it's a new trail or a well-trodden path at dawn, there's a zest to unearthing sights and sounds that you might not encounter with the chatter of companions or the distraction of a group's pace. The quiet courage in exploration can be as exhilarating as it is revealing about one's character.

At the same time, let's consider the sense of peace that accompanies solitary time in nature. The stress-dissolving quality of this peace cannot be overstated. It's akin to moving meditation, where each movement brings you closer to inner stillness, a contrast to the dynamic exertion of your body. This peace, this silence, is often where problem-solving thoughts arise and creative ideas take flight.

It's also worth noting the empowering realization that comes with knowing you're part of something larger. Surrounded by the age-old trees and mountains that have witnessed the arc of history, solitary workouts invite a humble acknowledgement of one's place in the grand tapestry of life. Such perspective is grounding and can evoke a tranquil sense of belonging to the world around you.

In conclusion, the experience of solo workouts is more than a mere exercise in physicality. It's a multifaceted pilgrimage into the self, set against the backdrop of the natural world. It's an intertwining of body, mind, and earth, each solo journey sowing seeds for growth—physical, mental, and spiritual. And remember, nature doesn't rush, yet everything is accomplished; in the end, so too are the achievements of your solitary sojourns, painted on the canvas of your spirit, one solo workout at a time.

Safety and Precautions for the Lone Adventurer

After embracing the beauty and resilience gleaned through the changing seasons and varied climates, one important consideration remains — venturing into nature's gym alone can be supremely rewarding, yet it comes with its own set of risks. When isolated from the buzz of a gym or absent the chatter of running partners, preparedness is your true companion. Sensible precautions pave the way to revel in solitude without compromising your safety.

First off, we must underscore the importance of planning. Before you head out, make sure someone knows where you're going and when you expect to return. It's easy to think you're just popping out for a quick jaunt, but nature has a way of serving up unexpected turns. A simple itinerary left with a friend can be a lifeline in rare cases of emergency.

Knowledge of your environment is equally important. Whether the mercury is swelling in summer or you're treading over winter's icy crust, understanding the elements and how they shift during your visit is crucial. This means studying the weather forecasts avidly and recognising when to don a waterproof shell or to pack an extra insulating layer.

Invest in a quality navigational tool like a GPS unit or a trusty, old-school compass which, unlike smartphones, doesn't fail when battery life wanes or when signal becomes a distant memory. Familiarising yourself with their usage before you go can save you more than just time; it can save your skin.

Speaking of gear, let's talk essentials. Whether it's a headlamp for those early morning runs, a whistle for attracting attention in an emergency, or a lightweight first aid kit for managing minor injuries, your equipment can be your salvation. Tailor your kit to the season and to the terrain — both can turn even the simplest outdoor workout into a demanding endeavour.

Hydration and nutrition are paramount, but they're often underestimated by solo adventurers — having enough water and energy-providing snacks can make the difference between a satisfying solo workout and a lethargic trudge back to safety. Even in winter, when thirst isn't as noticeable, your body loses water through breath and sweat. It's a balance; you'll need to carry enough but also manage your resources wisely.

Your own body can send out an SOS, and it's imperative you listen. Watch for signs of trouble like dizzy spells, excessive sweating, or the silence of your own breath in the cold. Pushing the envelope is one thing; tearing it apart is another. It's not defeat to turn back — it's intelligence.

Educate yourself on basic first aid and know how to address common issues that can arise when exercising outdoors. This includes anything from treating blisters to recognising the early symptoms of hypothermia. A good rule of thumb — practice addressing these conditions at home, because in the wild, there's no room for guesswork or learning on the fly.

In certain areas, wildlife can pose its own set of risks. Understanding which creatures share your environment and knowing what to do during encounters are both inaugural elements to your safety regime. Learn how to secure your food if you're venturing into areas where bears might roam, and become familiar with local snake species to differentiate between the harmless and the hazardous.

Moreover, always weigh the risks of the outdoor activities you choose to do alone. While it's vital to push boundaries to grow, some pursuits are best reserved for when you have company. Think critically about whether that solo rock climb or ice trek is wise without backup. There are plenty of rewarding ways to push your limits while still maintaining a margin of safety.

Learning to assess risks comes with experience, and there's no better teacher than nature herself. Start with smaller solo ventures and gradually progress to more demanding ones as you solidify your survival skills and deepen your understanding of your own limits and comfort zones within nature's embrace.

Finally, embrace technology, but don't become dependent on it. Battery packs can be a boon, but they're useless if wet or damaged. Understand that while a phone might help in an emergency, your best tools are your preparedness and wits. Have an emergency plan that doesn't involve waiting for a rescue that might be delayed or might never come.

Putting safety first doesn't mean dulling the thrill of adventure — it simply ensures that you can keep coming back to the environments that challenge and invigorate you. Taking on nature's gym alone is not about courting danger, but about knowing the dance steps well enough to glide through it with respect and readiness.

Once you're rooted in these practices, you'll find a harmony in solitude that complements the chorus of the outdoors. Every solo stride, swim, or climb will bind you more closely to the rhythms of the earth and the pulse of your own life. In times of solitude, that connection turns deeply personal and profoundly empowering. It's just you, the wide open, and the boundless potential of both.

Remember, the solo adventurer is never truly alone. Guardianship from danger often lies in the tools they carry, the knowledge they harness, and the intuition they fine-tune. Equipped with these, the solitary explorer isn't just as safe as those in a crowd — in many cases, they're better prepared, more attuned to their surroundings, and ready to reap the unique rewards that await when you step into nature's gym alone.

Chapter 14:
Group Dynamics: Social Sweat Sessions

A s we segue from the introspective journey of solo endeavours explored previously, we pivot to the undeniable energy and camaraderie found in group dynamics. Imagine the pulse-raising hustle of a team sport, the synchronicity of a cycling pack cutting through the morning mist, or the echo of laughter intertwined with the rhythmic thud of hiking boots on forest trails. Social sweat sessions are not just about elevating our heart rates together; they're a masterclass in human connection, weaving a tapestry of shared endeavors—a silent nod to the fact that we're all in this together. These communal acts of wellness embrace the essence of outdoor fellowship, where encouragement roars louder than any wind and success sweats from every pore, binding us in mutual respect for each other and our surroundings. There's a raw joy found in collective exertion—or simply in the stride of companionable silence—that reminds us that while nature doesn't discriminate, it certainly electrifies when we unite under its vast, open skies.

Organising Group Activities: From Hiking to Team Sports

We've braced ourselves against the elements, revelled in the changing of seasons, and now, let's gather our mates for something that can at times seem a bit more daunting than the most challenging trail or the steepest hill: organising group activities. Whether it's rambling through verdant woodlands or getting competitive in a friendly game of outdoor football, the benefits of group exercise are boundless. It's not just about the physical perk; it's the camaraderie, the shared memories, the burst of hearty laughter after someone's scenic tumble.

Organising a hike, to start off, isn't just plotting a route on a map. It's coordinating schedules, gauging everyone's fitness levels and interests, and ensuring you've all got the right kit. There's something deeply satisfying about leading a well-prepared group through the winding trails. The beauty of hiking in a group lies in the shared experience - the collective 'oohs' and 'aahs' as you crest a hill to reveal the landscape beyond, or the collective sighs of relief as you find a perfect spot for a midday picnic.

When it's not just walking but hiking is what tickles your fancy, remember it's a different game. Terrain dictates, and so does weather. You'll need to consider the pace – a balance between the thrill of a challenge and the assurance that no one is left huffing and puffing too far behind. It's about inclusivity, knowing when to take a break, when to push on, and when to simply stop and soak in the view.

Now let's swing the compass towards team sports. Football, rugby, cricket, or even a less traditional but highly fun round of ultimate frisbee – the options are endless. The key is in understanding what strikes a chord with the group. Some might find the idea of a friendly match invigorating; for others, it's the social interaction after the game that's the draw. Here, leadership means more than being the captain; it's rallying the troops, organising the location and equipment, and ensuring everyone walks off the pitch with lifted spirits, win or lose.

A gentle reminder: don't let organisation become a byword for military precision that drains the fun out of the endeavour. Flexibility is as significant as planning. When someone's late, or the weather throws a curveball, that's when the true spirit of group outdoorsmanship comes to the fore – adapting and finding joy in the unexpected. And it's alright to mix abilities; in fact, it's encouraged.

Those more experienced can lead the way and provide tips, whereas the novices can bring a fresh perspective and energy that can be downright infectious.

It's also important to remember that not every group outing needs to be an intense affair. There's beauty to be found in simplicity. A bird-watching amble or a leisurely cycle through the park allows for conversation and connection, while still reaping the benefits of outdoor activity.

Of course, there's always a bit of admin involved: make sure everyone knows the time and place, what to bring, and what to expect. Communication is your compass here; clear, concise, and considerate. Utilise group chats, social media or good old-fashioned phone calls to keep everyone in the loop. And gathering feedback after each outing will help fine-tune future ones. After all, it's everyone's adventure.

The feast after the famine, or rather, the socialising after the sweat, is as integral as the activity itself. Don't you skip it! Whether it's a picnic, a barbie, or just some snacks and drinks laid out on a blanket, this is where bonds are solidified, where the group stitches itself more tightly together.

And speaking of food – do cater to all dietary preferences. A sure-fire way to cast a pall over your post-activity camaraderie would be to have someone feel left out because there's nothing on the 'menu' they can enjoy. A little forethought goes a long way.

Then there's safety, an anchor of outdoor group activities. A well-stocked first aid kit, knowledge of CPR and basic first aid, and an action plan for potential emergencies can never be overstated. When you're in the great outdoors, preparedness is your best mate.

Remember to capture the moment too – photos or it didn't happen, right? But don't let snapping pictures overshadow the experience. Find the balance, savour the moment through your senses first, and the camera lens second.

Lastly, inclusivity extends to occasion as well. Birthdays, anniversaries, or simply the celebration of good weather – any reason's a good reason to bring people together. Sometimes, the best gatherings are impromptu, sparked by nothing more than a collective urge to get out and enjoy the day.

In the end, whether you've herded your mates up a hill or scored the winning goal in a friendly match, what lingers isn't the strain of the trek or the sweat of the sport – it's the laughter shared, the encouragement given, and the stories created. It's the realisation that, together, you've embraced the outdoors in a way that leaves you all a bit fitter, a lot happier, and craving the next escapade.

And while we're absorbed in the present, in these moments of shared exertion and elation, let's not forget to plan for the future. These activities, woven into our routines, become the bright threads in the fabric of our lives, adding texture and depth to our relationships and our memories.

So go on, be the instigator of adventure, the architect of outdoor escapades. Whether it's a quiet hike along a bubbling brook or an energising game on the grassy field, these group activities are where life's magic moments are minted. And isn't that what we're all after in the end – to feel alive, together, under the vast and beautiful sky?

The Bond of Shared Outdoor Experiences

Let's delve into a realm that transcends individual achievement and touches on the collective spirit – the bond formed through shared outdoor experiences. When we set out in groups, whether they're friends, family, or even strangers, there's a symphony of footsteps, a shared rhythm, that binds us. This bond serves as both a motivator and an enriching presence, adding depth to our encounters with the wild.

Picture the scene: a crisp morning, the sun barely peeping through the canopy of an ancient woodland, and a group of hikers, all different yet all connected by the simple act of moving through nature together. In these moments, words are often superfluous; it's the act of walking, climbing, or running side by side that forges our connection. Through mutual encouragement, we collectively push past perceived limits, discovering strength in togetherness.

Indeed, outdoor activities provide a unique stage for camaraderie to blossom. Be it paddling through meandering rivers or cycling winding trails, each person's energy radiates, affecting the collective experience. We learn about each other in a way that static environments rarely reveal: who sets a blistering pace, who has a keen eye for wildlife, or who can conjure laughter when the skies open and the rain pours down.

These shared experiences can be both intense and intimate, often leaving indelible memories. Take, for instance, the shared victory of reaching a mountain summit. It's not just the panorama that takes your breath away, but the shoulder-to-shoulder accomplishment, the joint surge of adrenaline and awe. This memory, shared amongst each other, becomes a story retold, strengthening bonds and inspiring future adventures.

Group activity in the outdoor realm also beckons the spirit of teaching and learning. Whether it's showing a novice the ropes of rock climbing or mastering the art of building a fire in damp conditions, shared knowledge becomes the currency of the wilderness. Each experience is an opportunity to grow and for expertise to ripple through the group, leaving everyone a tad wiser.

We cannot overlook the element of safety that comes with company. When we venture into less-trodden paths or undertake ambitious treks, having others to rely on is invaluable. It's a shared vigilance, a group commitment to each other's wellbeing. Should a mishap occur, there's solace in knowing that you are not alone and help is at hand.

Let's not forget the laughter and the stories that echo around the campfire. These are the soft glues that bind a group, the shared humor and narratives that weave through the group's collective memory. As we bask in the warmth of the fire and the company, we are reminded that joy is amplified when experienced with others.

Moreover, shared outdoor experiences can bridge gaps across generations and cultures. Whether it's a grandparent teaching a child to fish, or hikers from diverse backgrounds discovering common ground, the outdoors acts as a seamless integrator, dissolving barriers and fostering understanding.

It's these bonds, too, that can be channels of motivation. When our own resolve wavers, the support of a group can be the critical factor in taking that next step or paddling that extra mile. In truth, many have found their reservoirs of perseverance in the shared resolve of their companions.

While competition has its place, it's the spirit of inclusion and collective progress that often defines group dynamics outdoors. A trail run becomes less about who can finish first and more about ensuring everyone savors the journey. The group's pace organically adjusts so that all can participate and enjoy, embodying the true essence of teamwork.

The bond extends beyond the activity itself, often translating into committed environmental stewardship. As we grow closer to our fellow explorers, our collective connection to the environment deepens as well. We become advocates for the trails we've shared and the landscapes that have hosted our memories, fostering an ethic of preservation and respect.

In the shared silence of watching a sunrise or the hushed awe of encountering wildlife, there's a recognition of something greater than ourselves at play. It's these shared moments of wonder that can shift perspectives and create a powerful sense of oneness with the natural world.

When these shared journeys end, the bond often does not. The echoes of laughter, the triumphant whoops on summits, and the empathetic pats on the back transcend the confines of time and place. They become the threads of a tight-knit fabric, a community borne out of the shared outdoor experiences that continue to uplift and bind, long after the boots have been stored away.

In conclusion, it's clear that the richness of our encounters with nature isn't just shaped by the environment itself but is also deeply influenced by the company we keep. Together, we are more than solitary figures against the backdrop of the wild; we are a collective force, each individual's joy and triumph shared and magnified within the group. It's these experiences, these bonds, that illuminate the idea that the great outdoors is not simply a space to conquer or endure, but to share, cherish, and celebrate together.

Chapter 15:
Families Outdoors: Inclusive Fitness

With the echo of laughter in the air and the promise of adventure on the horizon, there's probably nothing more heartwarming than seeing families unite in the great outdoors, muddied boots and all. 'Families Outdoors: Inclusive Fitness' is the portal to a world where workouts aren't confined to the four walls of a gym, but rather sprawl under the vast canopy of the sky, inviting even the smallest tots to engage. It's all about creating experiences that cater to every family member—no one's left behind! Think games that double as agility training, nature walks sprinkled with bursts of playful sprints, or even the simple joy of a shared bike ride that caters to various fitness levels. It's the shared moments, the collective triumphs over a challenging trail, and the support that turns a routine into cherished memories. Here's where fitness isn't just about keeping active but about instilling a love for nature, teamwork, and the kind of exhilarating exhaustion that comes from a day well spent in each other's company. These are the days that seed a healthy lifestyle into the fabric of family life, ensuring the next generation rises both strong in body and deeply connected to the natural world around them.

Designing Family-Friendly Outdoor Activities

When we think about bringing the family together for some fresh air and sunlight, designing activities that cater to all ages can be a joyous puzzle. You see, the magic lies in creating moments that aren't just fun but are also enriching and adaptable to everyone's abilities. Let's delve into crafting outdoor activities that can galvanise the family unit into an adventure-loving troop.

Firstly, consider the varying energy levels and interests across your family. That bubbly toddler of yours might revel in the simplicity of chasing bubbles on the lawn, while your teenager could be yearning for something more engaging, like a friendly round of frisbee golf. It's all about the blend - incorporating elements of play that can spark joy in each member, ensuring no one is sidelined.

Identify your canvas – the great outdoors. Is it a park, a beach, your backyard, or a nearby trail? Every setting offers unique opportunities for activity and exploration. A beach day can transition from sandcastle building to a coastal walk with a scavenger hunt. Keep an eye out for different settings as they can provide natural inspiration for your next family outing.

Integration is key – think about activities that work well together. A picnic can be paired with cloud-gazing, or berry-picking can lead to an impromptu art session with nature's palette. This way, you're not just switching from one activity to another but creating a seamless and engaging experience for the family.

When planning activities, interactive elements that spark learning should be a priority. For instance, a simple hike becomes a mini-adventure when you turn it into a wildlife discovery walk, with the kids using their senses to look, listen, and learn about their natural surroundings. This not only makes the experience fun but also subtly educational.

Safety and preparation can never be overstated. Ensure you have a well-stocked first aid kit, make certain everyone's attired appropriately for the weather and terrain, and always have a plan if someone gets tired or the weather changes. Preparing ahead shows your family you've got everything under control, allowing them to fully immerse in the enjoyment of the day.

Variety spices up life as it does with family-friendly outdoor activities. Rotate your roster of activities to keep things fresh and exciting. One weekend might be dedicated to flying kites, while another could be focused on a friendly game of touch football. This rotation ensures everyone looks forward to discovering what's next.

Inclusivity is the golden rule. Design outings that allow for different skill sets and physical capabilities. Leisurely bike rides with options for various distances allow family members to choose their comfort levels without feeling pressured, and everyone ends up having a good time at their own pace.

The wonders of technology can be tapped into, rather than frowned upon. Organise a family photo challenge where each member uses their phone or camera to capture unique perspectives of nature, with the best photo earning the coveted spot on the family fridge. This embraces tech while promoting creativity and observation skills.

Don't shy away from the less-than-perfect weather days. Overcast can mean cooler temperatures for a hike, and a light drizzle can transform a regular walk into an exhilarating rain-soaked adventure, complete with puddle jumping competitions and the reward of warm drinks afterwards.

Sharing responsibilities heightens engagement. Assign tasks such as map reading or leading the walk to different family members, including the children. It not only teaches responsibility but also gives each person a sense of ownership in the family's activities.

Revisiting past successes can be a source of new fun. If a certain trail has brought joy before, go again but with a new twist – maybe this time, chart the path using nature's landmarks or a themed treasure hunt. Old favourites can provide comforting familiarity while the little changes keep the excitement alive.

A touch of spontaneity can often bring the most memorable experiences. Yes, planning is important, but so is the freedom to veer off the path for an impromptu game of hide and seek or to follow a curious butterfly's flight. Be flexible and open to the unplanned joys that nature often presents.

Fostering a spirit of adventure and discovery doesn't mean you have to climb the highest mountaintop. Sometimes, it's about seeing who can spot the most species of birds from your backyard. It's the keenness to explore and discover, more than the activity's grandeur, that imbues a sense of wonder in your family.

Finally, reflection is a splendid finale to any outdoor activity. Engage your family in a gentle discussion about what they enjoyed most, what they found challenging, and what they learned. These sharing sessions can reinforce positive experiences and provide insights for planning your next outing.

In conclusion, designing family-friendly outdoor activities calls for creativity, flexibility, and a willingness to embrace the quirks of varying preferences and abilities. It's about crafting an enriching tapestry of experiences where play, learning, and exploration intersect, leaving each family member with a treasure trove of outdoor memories.

Teaching Children to Love and Respect Nature

We find ourselves in an age where screens often eclipse the grandeur of the great outdoors, and despite our best intentions, our little ones might seem more enchanted by pixels than by ponds and pine forests. But within every child is an innate curiosity for the natural world, a curiosity that adults have the profound responsibility to nurture. By teaching children to love and respect nature we not only gift them a treasure trove of joy and wonder but also sow the seeds of stewardship for the environment that will last a lifetime.

Start by making the outdoors a regular part of family life. Whether it's summer's fiery energy you're soaking in, or the renewal of spring you're experiencing, outdoor activities should be as routine as bedtime stories. Adjust the frequency and intensity of these activities to suit the season—be it gentle walks in the autumn's crunchy leaves or building snowmen in winter's wonderland. Consistency here is key; you're establishing a rhythm, a pulse that beats in tune with nature's own.

As you dive into these seasonal wonders, turn each excursion into a learning experience. Teach them about the different types of foliage, the varying cloud formations, or why certain animals hibernate. Nature itself is a canvas for teaching; it's a living, breathing, ever-changing textbook that entices the senses and sharpens the mind.

Now, let's not shy away from the less-than-perfect weather. Did you know there's as much adventure in splashing through puddles as there is in summiting a sunny hill? It's time to embrace the rain, gear up, and show that every droplet of water has a story to tell. As those raindrops kiss the soil, share with your children the magic of the water cycle and life's dependence on this precious resource.

Beyond the science, imbue each adventure with respect for our natural world. Teach your children the principles of 'leave no trace', the art of interacting with wildlife without disturbance, and the importance of preserving the beauty we're privileged to enjoy. This harmonises beautifully with the ethos explored in the chapter on 'The Environmental Footprint of Fitness', wherein we pledge to limit our impact as we exercise through the seasons.

Engage their senses. Let them feel the bark, smell the roses, and hear the symphony of birdsong. These sensorial experiences forge an emotional connection—one much stronger than any lecture or admonishment could achieve.

Encourage stewardship through participation in conservation efforts. Perhaps there's a community garden that welcomes young green thumbs, or a stream clean-up that's looking for buckets—hands-on involvement like this reinforces the message that we all have a part to play in the well-being of our environment.

Don't be afraid to let children take the lead sometimes. Allow them to plan the route for a hike, or decide which veggies to plant in the garden. When they're invested in the decision-making, their engagement skyrockets, weaving a stronger bond between them and the green world.

Remember, nature should also be about fun and freedom. Some days might be about structured learning, while others could simply be about unbridled play in the great outdoors. Let them run wild—sometimes it's in the chaos of play that the deepest love for nature is kindled.

As the seasons change, as illustrated in the earlier chapters, ensure that adaptability is a lesson taught not just practically but emotionally as well. Children should understand that nature's gym doesn't close; it merely adapts and transforms, offering new and exciting ways to engage with the environment—whether it be skiing through snow or autumn leaf collection.

Of course, we must also speak to their imaginations. Nurture the wonder of nature through storytelling and shared narratives of outdoor adventures. Whether it's recounting a family hike up a snow-capped mountain or a summer camping trip spent beneath the stars, stories have the power to make a love for nature infectious and exhilarating.

While teaching respect for nature, it's crucial to demonstrate equal respect for the child's pace and interests. Gentle encouragement goes a long way—never force or push too hard. Whether they take to the outdoors like a duck to water, or show mild interest that needs cultivating, patience pays in nurturing a lifelong love for the environment.

Intertwine sustainability into their everyday practices. Explain why we choose eco-friendly gear, outlined in the efficient packing chapter, or why certain areas are off-limits to protect fragile ecosystems, as discussed in our section on 'Healing through Nature'. These are not just guidelines; they are actions that speak to the heart of preserving the earth for future generations.

Involve them in the broader community where the conversation about nurturing nature reverberates. There could be local clubs or national organisations dedicated to outdoor activities for children, offering structured programs and opportunities to socialize with likeminded peers—reinforcing their connection with nature through community spirit.

Finally, realise that this endeavour is a journey. Not every outing will be successful, not every nature fact will stick the first time, but persistence and enthusiasm are contagiously optimistic forces. The outdoors is a grand teacher—vast, forgiving, and wondrous. As guardians of these young minds, let's give the gift of the outdoors; let's craft childhoods rich with the verdant tones of the earth, for it is in these moments that the future custodians of our planet are born and bred.

Chapter 16:
City Meets Nature: Urban Outdoor Fitness

In any bustling metropolis, the notion of a close-knit tango between skyscrapers and spreading trees isn't far-fetched—it's happening in parks and greens across the city landscape. This blend of urban backdrop and nature's touch gives rise to a unique fitness vibe that distils the essence of both worlds. Imagine running along a smooth path, with the soft chorus of rustling leaves complimenting each stride, or practising Tai Chi as the sun rises, creating silhouettes against the serene cityscape. It's in these green pockets that, even in the heart of the city, you can whisk yourself away from the concrete jungle and immerse in an outdoor fitness regimen. This chapter is all about transforming city spaces into arenas for health, with routines that make every bench a chance for strength training and every clearing an opportunity to stretch under the urban canopy. It's here we reclaim our innate need for natural connection without ever having to leave the postcode—we simply step, jog or leap into the embrace of urban green spaces, letting the city's pulse fuel our workout, and nature's calm anchor our spirits.

Parks and Green Spaces: Lunges on the Lawn

Having explored the subtle art of adapting to the elements and finding serenity in solo routines, let's guide you closer to home—or, should I say, park—where green spaces beckon with open arms. These verdant sanctuaries present more than a patch of grass; they are symposiums for the body's dance with nature, equipped with nothing more than fervour, the open sky, and perhaps a sturdy pair of trainers.

So why choose a park when you have the comfort of a gym within arm's reach? The answers are multifold. Firstly, the canvas of green beneath your feet offers a natural cushioning, a respite for joints that pound against the unyielding brutality of concrete pavements and gym floors. The plush lawn underfoot is kinder, fostering a spring in your step as you lunge into the fitness world outside four walls.

Then, let's not overlook the symphony of our environment: birdsong, the whisper of leaves, and the occasional rustle of small fauna. Amidst this confluence of natural sounds, your workout attunes to a different rhythm, steering clear of the mechanical monotony of a treadmill's hum or the clatter of weights. The park is not silent; it is vibrantly alive.

Spatial freedom in a park is yet another gift. Without the confines of gym machinery, one's body becomes the spectacle of strength and agility, lunging forward, squatting, or gracefully transitioning into a warrior pose with room for sweeping movements. This freedom of space acts not just as a physical liberator, but it also unchains the mind, allowing creativity in exercise to flourish.

Breathing is never quite the same in the outdoors. Fresh, oxygen-rich air is synonymous with vitality, and when you inhale deeply amidst the greenery, you enrich your cells, amplify energy levels, and consequently, enhance performance. As you draw lungfuls of air, think of it as the most organic performance enhancer you could employ—courtesy of the park itself.

However, let's not shy away from the inherent unevenness the earth presents. This terrain, with its gradients and textures, proffers an intrinsic resistance and complexity to workouts. Each lunge and jump tests balance and engages core stability. Green spaces invite you to dance within their contours, promising a more wholesome workout every time.

Consider the psychological boons too. A park presents a fluid canvas where the moods of nature change from dawn to dusk, from one season to the next. This constant evolution imbues a dynamism to your workouts, ensuring that no two days in nature's gym are ever identical. It's hard to grow stale when each day's setting sun casts a new light on your exercise regime.

When we lunge in the lawn, engaging our thigh muscles, we can't ignore the parallel we draw with the growth around us. Just as the grass reaches for the sun, we stretch to meet our goals. Our bodies in motion emulate the natural growth that surrounds us—a synergy of existence.

Parks also champion the social aspects of fitness. While our journey can be solitary, the open lawn is often a community space where motivation is ripe for the picking. One can join impromptu fitness groups or even encourage a passerby to share a series of stretches. It's this opportunity for unexpected camaraderie that enriches our workout experience.

And then there's the warmth of the sun or occasionally the briskness of a surprise drizzle—well, aren't those part of the grand exercise experience? These elements bring their therapeutic touch to the equation, with sunlight providing a dose of Vitamin D and the rain, a refreshing cleanse. Our health isn't simply a product of physical strain but the environmental embrace as well.

Does all this talk about outdoor activity mean waving goodbye to your gym membership? Not at all. It's about balance, understanding that sometimes the best gym is the one without a roof, where your fitness pal is the towering oak and your instructor the unpredictable breezes that challenge your balance.

As for those necessary lunges on the lawn, they foster a connection with the earth that's visceral. With every lunge, every drop of sweat that anoints the grass, you're not just working out; you're participating in a rite as old as life itself—the rite of living beings moving under the sky, unbounded.

Sure, you might find yourself occasionally dodging a meandering beetle or pausing as toddlers career through your space—and that's perfectly alright. These gentle interruptions are reminders that you're part of something larger, an ecosystem where taking turns and sharing space come naturally.

To cap it all off, embracing parks for your fitness regimen is a nod to ecological mindfulness. By utilizing these communal spaces for health, we eschew the energy-intensive setup of gyms, reduce our carbon footprint, and reconnect with the core ethos of wellness—that it flows from and through nature.

Now, having painted this picture of lunges and liberty, of green canvases waiting to play host to your next workout, the park gates beckon. Go, explore, and discover your fitness amidst the harmonious concert of the great outdoors. After all, nature has a marvellous reputation—it never lets down those willing to lace up and step into its embrace.

When Nature Calls: Escaping the Concrete Jungle

Think about it — you're cooped up in cubicles, stuck in traffic jams, and suffocated by cityscapes so often you've almost accepted it as the norm. But there's that niggling, persistent urge, a subconscious whisper promising respite and peace, telling you to break free. You see, when nature beckons, it's worth heeding its call, trading the grey for green, the sounds of car horns for chirping birds, and the constricting walls for expansive skies.

Escaping the concrete jungle isn't just a luxury; it's a necessity for body and soul alike. But where to start? The key is to find pockets of nature nestled in your urban environment. It's often as simple as aiming for that leafy park you pass on your commute or the river trail you've heard about from a colleague. Allocate time in your weekly routine specifically for outdoor endeavors. You'll be surprised how this investment pays dividends in serenity and vitality.

Enticing as it may be, the challenge is often just stepping out the door. The city's convenience can be a double-edged sword, providing comfort while also stifling our inborn need for natural connection. Counteract this by setting tangible and regular outdoor objectives. Perhaps plan to jog through your local park three times a week or have a weekend picnic with friends. These commitments encourage you to step outside the city's steel embrace and into nature's nurturing arms.

Admittedly, the initial transition from artificial lighting and climate control to the unpredictable outdoors can be quite jarring. Fear not; you'll soon acclimate. Start small with strolls and gradually increase to hikes or other activities. The varied textures underfoot, the wind rustling through the trees, the unexpected downpours—they serve to remind us that being alive is a sensory experience.

For many city dwellers, the thought of nature calls to mind far-off mountains and untouched wilderness. They forget that nature is all around us, even in the heart of the metropolis. Spotting wildlife in an urban setting is especially thrilling. Birds, squirrels, and other creatures are adept urbanites. Observing them is a step towards re-engaging with the ecosystem you're a part of.

Now, here's the selling point: parks and green spaces in cities aren't just about aesthetics; they're your open air gyms. Exercise, when combined with fresh air and natural surroundings, can be significantly more effective in reducing stress than an indoor gym could ever hope to be. Whether it's yoga beneath a tree-canopy or bodyweight exercises on grassy knolls, the outdoor setting adds an invaluable dimension to your training.

Consider cycling or walking part of your commute. It injects a daily dose of outdoor time and also has a profound effect on your carbon footprint. In fact, consider any trip outside an opportunity to explore. Those errands you run? Turn them into mini expeditions. This practice begins to blur the lines between routine city life and the adventure of the outdoors.

Weekends are golden tickets for intensive escapades. Plan day trips to nearby nature reserves, forest trails, or coastal paths. These brief forays can be transformative, offering perspective and a great dose of high-quality air—proven to enhance lung function and, in turn, your overall exercise capacity.

Seasonal changes, which in the city can go unnoticed, become events to celebrate. The eruption of blossoms in spring, the shade provided by full green canopies in summer, the dazzling colors of autumn leaves, and even the stark beauty of bare winter branches offer a way to track time more richly than just by calendar and clock.

Urban community gardens are another secret weapon when you're needing a nature fix. Participating in gardening gets you hands-deep in the earth—quite literally grounding. There's something viscerally satisfying about nurturing growth, be it a plant or your own physical fitness. Plus, these spaces often create micro-communities, fostering social interactions bonded by a love of greenery.

If outdoor alone time is what you crave, understand that it is not just okay but often necessary. It's introspection in motion. Whether you're jogging, sitting, or just ambling, being solo in a natural space allows for a dialogue with oneself that's more revealing and more rewarding than in any enclosed space.

Don't let the urban sprawl deceive you; escapism is achievable. Start bringing living plants into your home. They improve air quality and mental health. Their presence can be a constant reminder of the world beyond concrete, waiting to be explored. You'll notice that even domesticated nature has a positive effect on your indoor environments, hinting at the potential of the outdoors.

We sometimesforget the simple truth: When it comes to boosting our well-being, a dose of nature is unparalleled. It's not just about fresh air; it's about reconnection. It's about tapping into the rhythm of life that the city beat often drowns out. So next time you feel hemmed in by the high rises, respond to that primal call. Step outside and take in the stretch of the sky, the grounding earth beneath your feet, the life that teems all around, and remember — this, too, is where you belong.

Plan ahead but be flexible. Weather changes swiftly and city environments can be fickle places. A spontaneous downpour can turn a planned workout into a dash for cover, and that's okay. Adaptability is key. The ability to switch gears and embrace the unexpected will not only serve you well in maintaining a nature-focused regimen but also in life.

Lastly, while you make these escapes, always remember to respect the areas you visit. Preserve the green sanctuaries within your city by following leave-no-trace principles and advocating for their care. These spaces are lifelines, not just for you, but for the community. When you care for them, you fortify that bridge between the city and the natural world. Now, pull on those trainers, step out the door, and let nature's revitalising call lead you to the tranquility and the adventure that await just beyond the concrete jungle.

Chapter 17:
Wild and Free: Exploring Remote Landscapes

Winding down the foot-worn path of urban workouts, we step into the vast expanse of remote landscapes with a heart full of yearning for the untamed wilds. Venturing beyond the comforting echoes of city life, there's an alluring call to the wild that's impossible to ignore when you're seeking to reconnect with your primitive self. Exploring these far-flung realms isn't just a stroll in the park; it's an intimate dance with nature herself, where every step is an orchestration of challenge and discovery, and the only audience is the rustling leaves and distant peaks. Whether it's the unyielding terrain that tests your physical prowess or the silence of the hinterlands that soothes your urban-weary soul, these havens of solitude serve as the ultimate playgrounds for the intrepid. As you trace the contours of these untrodden lands, you're not just trekking across the earth; you're charting a map of your inner strengths, navigating through brushstrokes of awe-inspiring scenery that can't be found within the confines of any gym. It's here, amidst the whispering grasses and towering ridges, that we uncover the purest forms of fitness and wellbeing—unhindered, unbounded, and unmistakably wild.

Off the Beaten Path: Planning Your Adventure

Imagine uncovering hidden trails and untouched landscapes where each step brings a sense of discovery. Such is the essence of going off the beaten path - a route less frequented but rich in secret splendour.

Venturing into the unknown requires not just a sturdy pair of boots and an adventurer's heart, but also methodical planning to ensure your endeavour is both stimulating and secure.

So, how does one plan an adventure away from the well-trodden trail? Step one is all about research. You'll want to spend time poring over maps – both digital and paper. Get familiar with the terrain, noting key landmarks and potential water sources. Understanding topography can be the difference between a delightful detour and an unwanted marathon.

Next up: gear. What you pack is critical to the success of your off-grid foray. You'll need the right equipment — something durable yet lightweight, to strike that delicate balance between preparedness and agility. From the correct shoes to cater to the terrain, to multifunctional tools that don't weigh you down, every item must earn its place in your backpack.

Considering the more unpredictable elements of nature, it's prudent to prepare for all weathers. Layering is key – you want to be as comfortable sweating up a hill as you are observing a starlit sky when the temperature drops. And don't forget a hardy, waterproof shell; hostile weather waits for no man, so best be ready for any sudden changes.

Communication is vital, too. While the point of going off the beaten path is to disconnect, you also won't want to be incommunicado in case you require assistance. A charged phone in a waterproof casing, a signal mirror, and perhaps a personal locator beacon should be part of your inventory. Leave a route plan with someone trustworthy; it's a safety net you shouldn't overlook.

There's also great joy in recruiting a like-minded companion. Not only does it offer the reassurance of having someone to rely on in the backcountry, but experiences shared are often the richest. Finding someone who matches your pace and enthusiasm for the natural world can elevate your adventure exponentially.

Let's talk sustenance. While you'll be nourished by the raw beauty of nature's gym, your body will need fuel. Pack high-energy snacks that don't spoil easily and consider water purification methods such as tablets or filters. Keeping hydrated and energised is as crucial as a good pair of hiking boots.

Now, onto pace. It's tempting to dash into the wilderness with all the exuberance of a child at play, but pacing is paramount. Know your limits and conserve energy; the goal is to enjoy the terrain, not just endure it. Your journey into the wild is more marathon than sprint, meant to be savoured with each step, not raced through to a finish line.

If your path is taking you through unfamiliar or particularly rugged territory, consider hiring a guide. They can offer expertise and local knowledge that could make your journey safer and more insightful, showing you secrets of the land you might otherwise have missed.

When you're deep in the embrace of nature, far from the chatter of society, and the only sounds are your breath and the chorus of the wild, you'll feel it. That profound connection to the earth, that pure sense of being alive. Whether it's the whisper of the trees, the call of a far-off bird, or the symmetry of the stones beneath your feet, the language of the natural world is sublime.

And when night falls, respect its dominion. A good tent or shelter is your sanctuary in the wilderness. Make sure you're well-practised in setting it up and taking it down so when fatigue sets in, your refuge is but a few minutes away. Sleep is critical – it's where the body and mind restore, readying themselves for a new day's adventure.

Safety should never be compromised for the sake of thrill. A comprehensive first-aid kit is a weight worth its gold, and understanding basic survival skills is essential. Knowing how to signal for help, start a fire, or navigate by the stars are not merely romantic notions of adventure — they could very well save your life.

Documenting your journey can also be incredibly rewarding. Whether through a written journal, photographs, or sketches, preserve the memory of the land through your unique perspective. Not only will you have personal mementoes, but you'll capture the essence of places few have seen, let alone remembered with such care.

Importantly, tread lightly. The ethics of leave-no-trace should be deeply ingrained in every adventurer's creed. We're but temporary guests in nature's house, so let's show the host the respect it deserves. Keep to existing trails where they exist, avoid disrupting wildlife, and carry out everything you bring in.

Finally, don't forget the most critical tool of all — instinct. Often, it's the soft nudge within that guides us through the path less followed. Trust in it, as it's the same primal instinct that has led explorers through the ages to discover the incredible wonders our world has to behold.

Now, with the maps studied, the gear packed, and the spirit willing, your journey awaits. May the path you choose bring the wonders of nature alive for you, in all its uncharted glory. Your adventure, meticulously planned, yet peppered with the unknown, will, no doubt, become a chapter in your life's rich tapestry that's spoken about for years to come.

The Draw of the Wilderness: Why We Seek Solitude

After exploring how nature can augment our physical conditioning, it's time to delve into a more introspective venture—the sometimes intangible, yet undeniable pull towards the wild expanses that lies within many of us. Those silent, sprawling spaces where it's just us against the backdrop of nature's vast canvas. We crave these encounters, seem programmed to seek out these environments. But why is it that the wilderness beckons us into solitude?

Have you not felt the surge within, the yearning to detach from the buzz of gadgets and the hum of industry, and find yourself within the cradle of the natural world? There's clarity in solitude, found amongst trees that whisper legacies, and rivers that run with untamed purpose. You find a sense of peace that can often elude us in the gridlocked confines of the urban jungle.

An ancient part of us lingers that knows only the wilderness as home. On a primitive level, the open spaces challenge and accept us, test our capabilities, and teach resilience. Embracing this challenge, we tap into an elemental version of ourselves often obscured by day-to-day concerns and social masks.

Let's not overlook the tangible benefits solitude in the wilderness offers for mental health. In an age where mental clutter is the norm, the simplicity of a forest or mountain range acts as a natural detox for the mind. Nature doesn't rush; it moves, cycles, and evolves at a pace that teaches us to slow down and harmonise with life's rhythm. It's healing to simply be part of that, to exchange chaos for calm.

Going solo into the wilderness also promotes self-reliance. It's you who navigates the trails, you who sets up camp, and you who decides when to rest or move on. Each step taken is a reminder of your autonomy, each mile conquered, an affirmation of your independence. Ever heard the phrase 'I found myself in the wild'? There's profound truth there—in the quietude of open spaces, you're faced with your intrinsic self, unadorned and raw.

Solitude in the wild, naturally, gifts you quality time for introspection. Away from the incessant demands of society, you're free to ponder life's big questions, reassess personal goals, and realign your compass in a direction that speaks true to your desires and aspirations. The silent dialogue between the soul and the open sky often yields the most profound revelations.

Moreover, solitude engenders a unique appreciation for the wonders around us. Solo excursions intensify the senses—you hear every rustle, see every hue, and feel every breeze. Nature, undisturbed, unveils its grandeur to the solitary wanderer in awe-inspiring clarity. You treasure each encounter, from the majestic eagle soaring overhead to the fascinating dance of insects on a leaf.

Our innate biophilia, or love of life and the living world, plays its part, too. There's a bond between us and nature that goes beyond recreational enjoyment—a deep, perhaps even spiritual connection. Solitude amplifies this bond, allowing for a communion with the earth and its creatures that often eludes us in communal settings.

In a society where constant social interaction is often seen as an indicator of happiness, choosing solitude can be a radical act. You defy the societal pressure that equates alone time with loneliness, discovering instead that within solitude lies freedom—an escape from the influence of others' opinions, a break from comparison and competition.

There's also a certain romanticism attached to the wilderness that has captivated the human spirit for centuries. Think of the literary reverence given to untamed landscapes—the drama, the inspiration, the muse it serves for artists and poets. In solitude, we compose our own epic, with nature as our muse, our solitude the canvas.

Consider how the wilderness brings us back to basics too; it's a reality check, reminding us of the essential minimalism we are capable of—where needs overshadow wants, and where priorities attain clarity. This dramatic stripping away of the non-essential affords a purity of existence that's hard to replicate in our material-laden world.

Solitude in nature also serves as a meditation. In the silence of vast expanses, broken only by natural sounds, we ascertain a meditative state that rejuvenates the mind, body, and spirit. It's a salve unlike any other, applied liberally as you traverse the terrains that knew no architect but nature itself.

No denial should be made of the bravery that solitude demands. To step out alone into the wilderness takes courage. It defies our deep-seated fears of isolation and vulnerability. But facing these fears head-on not only builds character but erodes the insecurities that bind us. The wilderness is a proving ground for our spirit.

And yet, for some solitude is not a quest but an encounter. It finds us in moments when the expanse of the sky, or the rustling leaves, or the serene mountain vista meets us as we are, and whispers of a truth we all share, but often forget—the truth that we are a part of this great tapestry, not merely observers but woven in, intrinsic to the wild and beautiful art of nature itself.

Seeking solitude in the wilderness eventually leads to an appreciation of the interconnectedness of all things. As much as we appreciate the time spent alone, we return with a heightened sense of our role in the larger community—both human and ecological. We're reminded that our actions resonate beyond our immediate surroundings and that we have a responsibility to tread lightly upon this Earth that has graciously hosted our solitary journey.

And so, you see, the wilderness in its vast, unfathomable depths offers more than just a venue for escapism. It is a place for discovery, reflection, and growth. Those who venture into its embrace alone come back with more than they sought—fortified in spirit, clear of mind, and rich with the profound knowledge that in solitude, we find much more than ourselves; we find our place within the magnificence of life.

Chapter 18:
Nighttime in Nature's Gym

As dusk settles and the world quiets down, there's an enchanting transformation within nature's gym that offers a unique realm of adventure and tranquillity for those who dare to explore. Enveloped in the velvety cloak of night, every rustling leaf and whispering wind becomes a confidential dialogue between you and the wilderness. It's a time when your senses sharpen, and what seemed familiar by daylight now challenges you with new mystery and wonder. Discovering the nocturnal secrets of the outdoors isn't just about the thrill; it's about cultivating a profound connection with the environment. Safety is paramount under the cloak of darkness, but so is the exhilaration of navigating trails with only the moon as your spotlight. You'll find your night vision improves with every step, and your confidence grows with each adventure. So embrace the cool air, let the starlit sky be your canopy, and allow the symphony of the night to guide your journey – after all, nature's gym is open 24/7, and nighttime might just become your new prime time.

Beneath the Stars: Safe Nighttime Adventures

Picture this: the quiet hum of nocturnal wildlife, the rustling of leaves in a gentle night breeze, and above, a tapestry of stars blanketing the sky. Engaging in nighttime outdoor activities presents a unique charm, an engagement with nature that feels almost secretive, reserved for those who dare to step into the darkness. But the night, while enchanting, brings about its own set of challenges and requires a higher attention to safety.

The first rule of thumb for any after-dark adventure is visibility. When the sun dips below the horizon, every outdoor enthusiast should equip themselves with a dependable source of light. Head torches are a treasure for hands-free navigation and, unlike handheld torches, they allow for full engagement in activities such as night running or setting up a campsite. Also, consider wearing reflective clothing or accessories to ensure you're visible to others, particularly important if you're near roads or trails shared with cyclists.

Let's talk about the company. Venturing into the night solo can be thrilling but embarking with a friend or a group not only adds a layer of security but also offers a shared experience that can tighten bonds. If a lone wolf experience is what you're yearning for, always inform someone about your whereabouts and expected return time. This is crucial, as it allows for a swift response should you encounter any unforeseen issues.

Orientation under the night sky can be deceptive. Mastering the art of navigation with a compass and a detailed map is invaluable when you're exploring under the celestial dome. Even if you're familiar with the terrain, the night can play tricks on your senses, transforming well-known routes into unfamiliar terrain. So, keep your map and compass handy and know how to use them.

Familiarize yourself with the nocturnal creatures you might encounter. Most wildlife poses little threat to humans, but knowing you might cross paths with intriguing nocturnal creatures adds to the excitement. Denizens of the dark such as owls, foxes, and bats become your unlikely companions, so learning to recognize their sounds and behaviors enriches your night-time excursion.

Stay warm. As the night progresses, temperatures can plummet. Don't be deceived by a warm day; always pack extra layers so you can adjust as needed. This is crucial to avoiding hypothermia, which can creep up unexpectedly if you're sitting still admiring the stars or waiting for the meteor shower you've hiked out to watch. Noise levels are lower at night, too, which means your voice won't carry as far, highlighting the importance of staying within sight of your group or camp.

And speaking of meteor showers, aligning your outdoor activities with celestial events can be a stunning highlight. Whether it's a night hike to witness the Northern Lights, or finding the perfect spot to gaze at a lunar eclipse, the cosmos offer shows that no cinema can match.

Technology can be your ally in the darkness. While it's essential to disconnect from time to time, a fully charged mobile phone is a lifesaver in emergencies, especially with GPS capabilities. Downloading offline maps and investing in portable chargers can keep you connected when needed.

Food and drink take on even greater importance at night. It's easy to underestimate your body's needs when you're distracted by the exhilaration of the dark. Keep energy levels up with snacks, and hydrate well; the cool of the night might mean you don't feel thirsty, but your body is still losing fluid.

Let's not forget about the place we've come to savour. Leave no trace principles become even more pressing in the vulnerability of night. Minimize your impact, keep noise to a minimum, and pack out whatever you bring in. The stillness and purity of a night environment should be left as they are for the next set of wanderers.

Terrain can be trickier to navigate by night. Uneven paths, roots, and rocks become hazards. Slow down and take your time. There's no rush under the moon's watchful eye. Pick activities that match your night-time navigation skills and build on them progressively.

It's not just about safety, though. Nighttime activities offer a unique way to challenge your physical fitness, with reduced visibility demanding higher focus and balance. Your body works differently in the cool of the night, and adapting to this can boost your endurance in surprising ways.

As for mental resilience, there's something special about the stillness that envelops you under a night sky. It can be a meditative experience, allowing for deep introspection and a remarkable sense of peace. You'll find your senses heightened, attuning more acutely to every sound and movement. The night, indeed, can be a teacher guiding you towards greater mindfulness.

Camping overnight can extend your adventures and give you a full spectrum experience of the natural nocturnal world. Understanding how to set up a safe campsite, respecting wildlife, and managing fire safety are all part of this immersive adventure. Waking up to the first rays of dawn after a night well-spent outdoors is a joy unlike any other.

In the embrace of darkness, armed with knowledge and respect for the environment, you're set for a workout that stimulates not just the body but the soul. So go on, lace up those boots after sunset and take your place beneath the stars. Every step, every breath under the night sky is a reaffirmation of our incredible journey on this planet.

As you return from your nighttime exploration back to the lights and sounds of dawn or dusk, carry with you not just the memory of the stars but the knowledge that you've navigated the night with respect, caution, and an open heart. Until the next twilight beckons, rest well, for the night has its magic, its own rigorous training ground, and its lessons that linger long after the shadows have retreated.

The Quiet of the Night: A Different Sensory Experience

Slipping into the cloak of darkness, the world transforms. The hustle of daylight ebbs, making way for the calm symphony of nocturnal whispers. Nighttime in nature's gym isn't merely an absence of light; it's an entirely different arena where senses are heightened, and the very air around us seems to thrum with possibility.

Sounds become the leading characters in this new setting. Stripped of the dominant visual cues, our ears pick up the subtleties often missed during the day: the rustle of leaves as a night creature scurries by, the hooting of an owl echoing in the distance, or the rhythmic chorus of crickets. This acoustic landscape can become an unexpected soundtrack to our nocturnal exercises, enriching the experience with a dose of wild serenity.

Touch, too, is magnified under the moon's silver glow. The sudden rush of cool air against skin when emerging from the cover of trees, the texture of the earthy ground beneath feet, or the faint mist that envelops the body are all tactile reminders of nature's presence, wrapping around us in the gentlest of embraces.

Let's not forget the scents. Night air carries with it an aromatic tapestry woven from the earth's cooling soils and the release of blooms that prefer the moon's audience over the sun's. These fragrances provide a refreshing change from the often overpowering smells of day; they're subtle, yet they linger, weaving through each breath, invigorating the lungs and refreshing the soul.

If you feared losing sight itself, fret not. The eyes adjust—night vision may not be our strong suit but given time, the shades of darkness reveal shapes, movements, and a vague outline of the world. The night sky, a spectacle on its own, with constellations telling ancient stories, becomes a breathtaking canopy for fitness endeavours.

Working out at night offers opportunities for unique activities that just don't feel the same during the day. Imagine yoga under a sky punctuated by stars, your body moving in harmony with the universe. Think of trail running where every step is a trust exercise with nature, guided only by the staccato of your heartbeat and a narrow beam of light.

Here we are, in a world fundamentally the same as the daytime, but perceived through entirely different lenses—well, senses. It's the altered perception that turns a regular path into an adventure. So, let go of any need for the familiar. Embrace uncertainty as you explore this sensory playland. You'll find your body's responses intriguing, perhaps even surprising, as it adapts to the darkness.

Beyond enhancing senses, the night's quiet also offers psychological benefits. The solitude and peace are perfect for introspection or processing the day's events. As you jog, hike, or simply move through the moonlit landscape, you might find the quiet to be an excellent partner for unwinding and sorting through thoughts.

Of course, night encounters aren't without their practical considerations. Safety becomes paramount. Make sure you're equipped with the right gear: headlamps, reflective clothing, and perhaps a buddy to share in the nocturnal escapades. Safety aids in keeping your mind at ease and allows for a fuller, richer immersion into the nightly exploration.

Engaging in night activities also calls for adaptation. Slow down your activities to match the environment. There's no need to mimic the intensity or speed of daylight workouts; the night is not about setting records, it's about immersion, about moving in sync with the silky threads of darkness that dance around you.

The night beckons the brave, the curious, and the tranquil souls. It's a canvas expecting to be painted with the steps of those wanting to experience nature in its truest, most raw form. There's an unparalleled sense of freedom in embracing the outdoors without the sun's watchful eye, a liberation that can be profoundly empowering.

As the chapter of night unfolds, allow yourself to be led by intuition and the natural cues that emerge. It's okay to feel a bit disoriented or less surefooted—these moments push us to grow, to refine our balance and our movement. Nighttime outdoor pursuits aren't just about physical fitness but are also a journey towards internal strength and confidence.

Wary about taking the first step into the night? Start with a familiar trail, one well-trodden during the day. Your memory will serve you, lending confidence as your senses adjust. Gradually, as comfort grows, so will your boundary of exploration. Before long, the night will feel like an old friend rather than an uncharted territory.

In this otherworld, where starlight plays with shadows and the air caresses with unseen hands, fitness intertwines with the spirit of the wild. The quiet of the night: a sanctuary that tests, teaches, and tenderly guides us to a place where the senses reign supreme and the experience of nature is deep, visceral, and profound.

Plunge into the quiet of the night and rediscover the familiar world in a plethora of new, vibrant forms. Each step under the celestial dome contributes not just to your physical well-being but also to a sensory and spiritual richness that only the enveloping embrace of nighttime can bestow. So go ahead, step into the night's gym and witness your senses come alive in the hush that descends when the sun dips below the horizon. The quiet of the night awaits you — will you answer its call?

Chapter 19:
Mindfulness and Wellness in the Great Outdoors

As twilight fades into the calm of night, we turn our focus inwards, finding our breath rhythm echo the gentle rustle of leaves in *Mindfulness and Wellness in the Great Outdoors*. It's about cultivating a tranquility that's not just carried on the breeze but also emanates from within as we immerse ourselves in the stillness of nature. Draw a deep breath, feel your lungs expand, and let's slowly unwrap the art of syncing our inner peace with the world around us. Here, we're not just moving through the landscape; we're setting the stage for a deeper, more nourishing interaction with the elements. Dive into practices like outdoor yoga, which nourishes both the body and soul amidst the grandeur of the peaks or the serenity of a forest clearing. Here, every pose and stretch is an ode to the earth beneath us; every meditation becomes an intimate dialogue with our natural surroundings. This is where wellness transcends the physical - it's a holistic dance, a synergy that encompasses the boundless skies above and the sturdy ground below. Feel the gutsy wind, the sun's nurturing warmth, or the introspective grey of an overcast day; each holds a lesson in balance and harmony, inviting us into a state of mindful serenity that stands firm against life's relentless rhythm.

Breathing Exercises Amidst the Elements

Imagine standing on a soft forest floor, the air kissed with the scent of pine, your lungs filling with the earth's freshest oxygen. Here, amongst the dance of elements, lies an opportunity to rejuvenate not just through motion, but through the very act of breathing.

Breathing - it's instinctive, necessary, yet often overlooked in our fitness routines. When we step outdoors, the quality of air changes, and so does our connection to the breath. Allowing your lung to ride the waves of fresh outdoor air can add a new dimension to your well-being.

Consider the crispness of a spring morning and the gentle caress of a mild breeze. Such a backdrop calls for a breathwork regime that awakens your senses, mirroring the rebirth happening all around you. Try a series of deep inhales followed by slow, deliberate exhales, syncing each breath with the rise and fall of the sun to truly harness the energy of the season.

As the mercury rises and summer asserts itself, your breathing should adapt. Heat demands respect, and so shorter, more frequent breaths become the order of the day. It's the perfect time to draw energy from the fiery sun, using quick, energising breaths to fuel your pursuits and maintain a sense of coolness within.

Autumn brings about a measured approach, much like the steady descent of leaves from the trees. Your breathing can take on a rhythmic, calming pattern here. Seek a pace that harmonises with the occasionally gusty winds, strengthening your diaphragm and amplifying your sense of inner balance.

Winter's chill presents its unique challenge, with cold air often leading to tighter airways. Breathing exercises during this time should be warming and grounding. Paced breathing, where you count steadily during each inhale and exhale, can regulate your body's response to the cold and help insulate your core temperature.

That's not to say that the elements are always mild or accommodating. When rains lash, as they often do, let your breath patterns trace the rhythms of falling droplets. Use dynamic breathing techniques that harmonise with the soundscapes around you, filling your lungs with moisture-rich air that invigorates the senses.

Wind days bring their own thrill. Let the unpredictable gusts guide your breath – inhale as the breeze lifts, hold as it plateaus, and exhale as it dies down. This synchronisation not only strengthens your respiratory system but also instils a calm, centred state of mind.

Playing with temperatures is also rewarding. While the coolness of dawn prompts an inward, reflective breathing style, the heat of the midday might call for you to focus on the exhalation, ridding your body of built-up warmth and encouraging a sense of refreshment.

Remember, breathing in the great outdoors isn't just about the physical act. It's a full-sensory experience that binds you to your environment. Take time to notice the scents on the breeze, whether it's the salt from the ocean, the sweetness of blooming flowers, or the earthiness that comes after a bout of rain.

Even in urban settings, you can still find your breathing oasis. A park or a rooftop garden can provide the greenery necessary to filter the air, allowing for cleaner, deeper breaths. Witnessing the transition of light during sunset or sunrise in such spaces can inspire breaths that are both mindful and rejuvenating.

And what of snow and ice, you ask? Whether you're basking in the quietude of a snowfall or braving the bite of icy winds, your breathing exercises become a tool for endurance. Embrace the sharp inhalations and the misty exhales as badges of your resilience, and find your inner warmth through the rhythm of your breath.

Across all these exercises, consistency is key. Make breathing practice a regular part of your outdoor routine and notice how your lung capacity increases over time. Elevate each breath with intention and awareness to extract the full benefit from the very air you draw.

It's also worth considering the impact of altitude on your breathing. At higher elevations, the air is thinner, and each breath delivers less oxygen. In such places, engage in breathing patterns that maximise intake, and allow for frequent pauses to accommodate your body's acclimatisation to these new heights.

In the end, each breath taken amidst the elements is a step closer to a deeper attunement with nature. It's about finding that splendid harmony between the air around you and the life force within you. So the next time you lace up for an outdoor adventure, take a moment, fill your lungs, and let the elements teach you the ancient art of breathing – instinctive, nourishing, and beautifully vital.

Outdoor Yoga and Meditation: Finding Your Zen Zone

Amidst the immersive tapestry of sounds, sights, and scents that nature unfurls, there's hardly a greater stage for refining our mindfulness than the untamed outdoors. Imagine unfurling your yoga mat on a bed of soft grass, the sky's expanse above choreographing a dance of drifting clouds as your background. Outdoor yoga and meditation aren't just exercises in physicality; they're an exploration of the mind's frontiers, a quest for an inner stillness that mirrors the majestic calm of the natural world.

It's well-known how nature's tranquil settings can amplify the potency of meditation and yoga. The breathable fabric of fresh air, paired with the soft hum of forest life or the lullaby of waves, can facilitate deeper states of calm. When yoga poses stretch limbs and meditation clears the mind, the outdoor milieu enhances the experience, enabling practitioners to find their 'Zen Zone' in the harmony of open-air serenity.

To embark on this journey, one must first find a spot that feels like a natural extension of oneself. This means scouting beyond manicured lawns and flagged pavilions to quieter corners of parks or sequestered beaches where the kinetic hustle of daily life does not intrude. One's chosen refuge should be a place where interruptions are unlikely, a cradle for concentration and uninterrupted flow.

Once the physical stage is set, it's vital to anchor ourselves within the environment. Grounding exercises—feeling the earth beneath you, engaging all your senses to absorb the surroundings, can help attune your frequencies with the natural world. Incorporating outdoor elements into your practice can be transformative; sun salutations under the morning sun take on a poignant realism, and breathing practices align with the breeze's rhythm.

Outdoor meditation allows for a symphony of natural cues to guide your practice. Whether it's the rhythmic lapping of a lakeshore that becomes the focus for a mindfulness session or the intricate patterns of leaves that encourage visual meditation, these organic elements are dynamic aids in achieving mental clarity and emotional poise.

Weather conditions, too, play a decisive role. While a sunny day offers warmth and uplifting energy, an overcast sky can induce a poignant, reflective state conducive to deeper meditation. The key is to welcome the weather as a participant in your practice, letting it shape your experience without resistance.

When temperatures dip, this doesn't signal the end of outdoor sessions. On the contrary, crisp air can invigorate your senses and deepen your breathwork. The trick is to layer appropriately, allowing for warmth without restricting movement. An over-sized sweater, some warm leggings, or even a simple blanket for Savasana can make all the difference.

The melodic rise and fall of wind through the trees can offer a soundtrack to yoga and meditation. Let your breath sync with this natural ebb and flow, using gusts to guide your expansion and stillness for deeper introspection. The wind not only cools the skin but can also stimulate a fresh perspective, whisking away stagnant thoughts much like it scatters autumn leaves.

Ignoring the life cycle of nature would be a disservice to outdoor practice; the vibrant growth of spring can inspire renewal in your routine, while autumn's shedding process might echo in a mental letting-go of burdens. Aligning with nature's rhythms encourages a synchronicity that deepens the contemplative and restorative process.

The soundscape of your environment becomes a subtle guide during meditation. Whether it's the chorus of crickets as dusk falls or the distant cacophony of geese migrating overhead, these natural harmonies can be the metronome to your mindfulness, an echo of the planet's pulse within your own practice.

As dusk descends, the diurnal shift from daylight to twilight can be magical for yoga. Transitions between asanas might reflect the gentle fade of light, and the cooling air can draw sharper focus to your internal journey, cushioned by the velvet of nightfall. Outdoor yoga under an expansive canopy of stars adds an astronomical dimension, opening up vast spaces within and without.

There's an undeniable connection between yoga, meditation, and the land they're practised upon. Tread lightly, respecting your environment by embracing leave-no-trace principles, using sustainable yoga mats, and minimising disturbance to wildlife. This responsible approach ensures nature remains unfettered, a gift for future generations and a testament to mindfulness in action.

In moments of pause, look around and enshrine memories within your mind. The hues of autumn, the sparkle of a frost-covered landscape, the vibrant greenery of summer — these snapshots can be revisited during indoor practice, a mental portal to your Zen Zone when you can't step outside.

Don't shy away from the less conventional aspects of meditation either, such as walking meditations. Meander along a forest trail or a mountain path with conscious steps, allowing each footfall to be a reminder to stay present, to cherish the gentle dialogue between soul and soil. It's a perfect way to blend the art of motion with the stillness of meditation.

As this chapter closes, remember that the Zen Zone is not a distant, isolated point on a map. It's a tranquil state of mind that moves with you — unbounded by walls, always underfoot, and lingering on the fringes of your eyelids as they close in contemplative grace. Find it beneath the swaying boughs, on the sunbathed shore, amongst the whisking grasslands; find it wherever you open your heart to the wild embrace of nature. And there, in the outside classroom of countless lessons and boundless potential, keep finding that still point of the turning world.

Chapter 20:
Thrill-Seekers and Adrenaline Junkies

Now, let's shift gears and channel our inner daredevil, where the wild heartbeat of nature pushes the envelope of exhilaration. For the thrill-seekers and the adrenaline junkies, embracing the outdoors isn't just about a fresh workout setting; it's about fusing the rush of extreme sports with the raw beauty of nature. These audacious spirits aren't satisfied with the treadmills and weight racks; they're out scaling cragged peaks, surfing tempestuous waves, and tearing through backcountry on mountain bikes. And why? Because facing nature at its most intense is both humbling and empowering. It's this dance on the edge of risk and control where our mental fortitude is tested and our physical limits are defied. Yes, there's a fine line between recklessness and robust adventure—we respect that line. Safeguarding our wellbeing while courting the wild winds of thrill, that's where the heart of this chapter beats strongest. So, let's explore the structured chaos of storm-chasing surfers, high-altitude cyclists, and the myriad of outdoor pioneers who remind us that sometimes, to truly feel alive, we must daringly engage with the forces that make this planet remarkable.

Extreme Weather Sports: Safety and Thrills

Cast your imagination to the highest snow-capped peaks, the fiercest waves on a stormy coastline, or the barren expanses of a desert at the peak of summer heat. Extreme weather sports aren't for the faint of heart, but they offer an unparalleled rush for those who dare to face nature's most formidable moods. It's not just about the thrill, though. It's also a conversation with the elements, an elaborate dance where safety steps and preparation are your partners.

Think of outdoor enthusiasts who venture out when the wind howls, snow blinds, and sun scorches. They aren't reckless; they're calculated. The thrill in extreme weather sports hinges on the fine balance between calculated risk and safety measures. The first rule is respect – for the weather, the environment, and your personal limits. Ignoring any of these aspects can transform an adventure into a misadventure rather swiftly.

Weather predictions and readings are gospel in the realm of the extreme. Tapping into high-tech gear and traditional know-how to interpret the skies can make the difference between an exhilarating experience and a call for rescue. Before setting foot on the slope, in the wave, or on the trail, hours are spent studying patterns, knowing when to advance, and when to retreat to the warmth of a fire or shade of a cove.

Appropriate gear also becomes a non-negotiable investment. Think beyond aesthetics; what you wear and carry must serve a purpose – insulation, hydration, communication, or navigation. It's this equipment that stands as your first line of defense against the volatile touches of Mother Nature. The choice of wear isn't just a statement but a carefully chosen utility for the extreme sport you're engaging in, whether it's insulated wetsuits for cold water surfing or crampons that cut through the deceitful beauty of a glacial hike.

Training and physical preparedness align next. Your body is your most crucial gear in any extreme condition. It has to be finely tuned, like a well-oiled machine, ready to withstand pressure, cold, and fatigue. Training switches between endurance, strength, and technical skills, each as important as the other. Consider the ice-climber whose grip must remain firm despite the biting cold or the desert runner whose resilience is tested with each mirage that shimmers on the horizon.

Yet, the call of the wild can be a siren's song – tempting but dangerous. Learning the art of self-rescue and first aid is vital, a skill set that one hopes never to employ but takes comfort in possessing. Resilience isn't just about enduring but also about knowing how to patch up a wound, set up an impromptu shelter, or signal for help when all the planning fails to account for the unforeseeable.

Extreme weather sports come with a silent clause: the guarantee of unpredictability. One day is different from the next, and flexibility becomes your best strategy. It's why a snowboarder might wake before dawn to assess a slope or a sandboarder might retreat into the dunes when the wind shifts. It's not a retreat, but a tactical withdrawal, knowing that the environment commands the final say.

In the face of such formidable forces, camaraderie often becomes as crucial as the gear you wear. A trustworthy team can be the difference between success and failure. It's about more than simply sharing the thrill; it's about watching out for one another, sharing knowledge, and skills, and being the voice of reason when adrenaline threatens to cloud judgment.

Embracing the ethos of leave no trace is also ingrained deep within the heart of the extreme sports enthusiast. They venture out, not to conquer but to become a small, fleeting part of the landscape. The mark left on their souls by nature's power is deep, yet they strive to ensure their physical footprint is minimal.

And then there's the aftermath of the adventure, the serene aftermath where stories are shared, photos are scrutinised, and the experience is relived. It's a time to reflect on what the mountains taught, how the waves spoke, or the way the desert's silence echoed with life. This reflective practice allows for growth and understanding and prepares the mind and body for the next encounter with the extreme.

The pull of extreme weather sports is undeniable for those seeking to push themselves beyond their comfort zones. It's a transformative journey that reshapes one's perspective on potential, resilience, and life itself. And while the pursuit of thrills is a powerful draw, it's matched by an equal commitment to safety, preservation, and respect for the raw, untempered beauty of our environment.

So, when you next watch the storm clouds gather with an impish sparkle in your eye, remember that the dance with extreme weather isn't just about the rush. It's a symbiotic partnership with the elements, one where caution, respect, and awe lead the steps. Here lies the truest form of thrill – the thrill of becoming one with the tempest while holding the line, securely tethered to safety and the respect for the power of nature.

May your adventures be many, your stories epic, and your respect for the vast playground of nature deep and unyielding. Here's to the thrill seekers who look beyond the fury of the elements and see a canvas for an exhilarating, life-affirming masterpiece. Just remember, the paintbrush comes with responsibilities, and the masterpiece you create should leave no scars on the canvas that is our wild, wondrous world.

Pushing Personal Limits: Healthy Risk-Taking Within these pages, stories have been woven of embracing nature's gym throughout every season. Now, let's pivot to a topic buzzing with invigoration— healthy risk-taking. When you think about pushing your personal boundaries, it's not just about the adrenaline rush. It's about discovering more of who you are and what you're capable of.

Healthy risk-taking is a nuanced dance between the familiar and the unknown. It's the bold step of entering a longer race, the decision to hike further or the resolve to lift the heavier weight. These are calculated risks; you're not jumping into unknown waters without first learning how to swim. You've prepared, you've trained, and now you're set to stretch the limits just a tad more.

Why take risks, you might ask? Our nature cravings are not just for the beauty of the green leaves or the softness of the snowflakes; they yearn for the feeling of achievement when we surpass our known abilities. To engage in an outdoor activity that tests our limits gently is to be alive and in touch with our innate human desire for growth.

Let's be clear: this isn't about being reckless. Each venture into the zone of proximal development requires forethought. It's essential to understand the weather's impact, the terrain's challenge, and one's physical condition before taking a step. Stepping out of your comfort zone is not about abandoning caution but expanding it in service of personal growth.

Assessing the risks involved is the first order of business. Whether you're a seasoned outdoor enthusiast or a newcomer, it's crucial to research, plan, and execute within reasonable safety margins. For instance, if snow sports enthral you, making your first foray onto the slopes should come after lessons and under watchful eyes.

Risk-taking is also deeply personal. Your mountain might be another person's molehill. The key is not to compare but to focus on what makes your heart race a little faster. Maybe it's trading the treadmill for a trail run or swapping the swimming pool for open water. These healthy risks should be embraced as steps towards a more robust self.

It's equally important to appreciate the role of patience. Sometimes risks are calculated over months, not moments. Preparing to climb a new peak or to cycle a century does not happen overnight. It demands consistent effort and incremental increases in intensity or duration. This slow pushing of boundaries is often where the true magic of transformation occurs.

Beyond the planning and physical training, there's a mental aspect of risk-taking that we can't ignore. Preparing your mind for the discomfort of new challenges is as crucial as pre-conditioning your body. Visualisation techniques, goal setting, and positive self-talk are the silent allies of the outdoor warrior who seeks healthy risk-taking.

Shared experiences in risk-taking can amplify benefits, too. When you pair up with like-minded folks, you forge a collective momentum. It's about support, shared knowledge, and sometimes, that sheer push from someone saying, "You've got this!" Being part of a group can ease the intimidation of risk-taking, making the leap more manageable.

Yet, the rewards of taking risks are intimate and alluring. The surge of endorphins when you reach a summit or complete a daunting paddle is transformative. It whispers to the essence of your being that you can do more, be more. The self-knowledge gained from these experiences, the understanding of your resilience—these are treasures unearthed in the great outdoors.

Knowing the balance between pushing too far and not enough is a delicate art. It's wise to listen to one's intuition and body signals. Pain, strain, or sheer exhaustion are not badges of honour but signs to reassess and calibrate. Healthy risk-taking means knowing when to press forward and when to retreat and try another day.

As you consider where to nudge your boundaries next, remember that nature is a forgiving gym. It challenges you with hills and thrills but also teaches you the grace of recovery and rest. After a hard-earned risk, returning to the embrace of a quieter, gentler activity is not an admission of defeat but a part of the cycle of growth.

Documentation of your risks and rewards can be a powerful tool. Whether through journaling your outdoor endeavors or capturing moments with a camera, these records serve as reminders of where you've been and markers for future adventures. They're proof of your capacity to evolve and expand your horizons.

In the end, healthy risk-taking is about respecting your limitations while gently prodding them. It's about honouring how far you've come and yearning for the paths you've yet to tread. And as you lace up your boots, strap on your helmet, or grip your oars, remember that it's not just the destination that counts—it's the thrill of the journey and the pride of knowing you dared to dance with risk and emerged stronger, wiser, and more alive.

Embrace this facet of nature's lessons; it's a realm where rewards are not in medals or podiums, but in the widened eyes of your spirit, reflecting the vastness of the outdoor wonders you dared to explore. Pushing personal limits, after all, is less about outdoors prowess and more about the unfolding map of your untapped potential.

Chapter 21:
Healing through Nature

After exploring the adrenaline-fuelled heights of extreme sports, let's shift our focus to a transformative aspect that's equally exhilarating—the restorative embrace of the Great Outdoors. Imagine a place where the air is a symphony of earthy scents, the landscapes a palette of nurturing colours, and the ambiance a gentle caress to both body and soul. This isn't just a scene set for serenity; it's a potent remedy and a crucible for recovery. Immersing oneself in green spaces isn't merely a retreat from the cacophony of urban life; it's an invitation to participate in a natural healing process. Through each breath in a forest or a stroll by a babbling brook, nature incrementally weaves its magic, knitting together the frayed edges of our well-being. Think of it not as a passive experience, but as an active engagement where each step taken outdoors is a step towards convalescence. It's in these therapeutic environments that we unearth resilience, discover tranquility, and facilitate both physical and emotional healing. As we delve into the nurturing arms of nature, remember that recovery, much like the growth of the mightiest oak, starts with the smallest seed—nourished by the soil of patience and the sunlight of persistence.

Green Spaces as Therapeutic Environments

Imagine stepping onto a lush expanse of grass, the chirping of birds serenading your presence, leaves whispering secrets to the wind. This isn't just an escape; it's an immersion into a healing sanctuary carved by nature's own hands. For countless individuals, green spaces serve as more than mere visual delights—they're wellness oases promising restoration and tranquillity. In our collective pursuit of health, these natural backdrops aren't mere set pieces but vital partners in our journey.

Consider the gentle pace of a garden stroll, a sublime contrast to the relentless tempo of urban existence. In the heart of nature, our breath deepens, stress recedes, and the heart finds its rhythm in harmony with the rustling foliage. Scientific studies are no stranger to these effects, repeatedly drawing conclusions that nod to nature as a conduit for better mental health. Anxiety, depression, and that sense of being perpetually 'on edge'—they all seem to dissipate as one is enveloped by a canopy of green.

And it's not only our minds that reap these rewards. Our bodies respond with gratitude to time spent in green spaces. From improved cardiovascular health to strengthened immune systems, the physical benefits of integrating nature into one's fitness routine are compelling. Workout turns to play, exertion intertwines with exploration, and through each leap and bound, one's wellbeing soars.

Consider the therapeutic effect of textures underhand—the tactile joy of a dew-kissed leaf or the roughness of tree bark. Visually, there's much to enamour the eyes too: the multiplicity of hues, the dance of shadows and light, and the gentle decay that remind us of life's cycles. All of these elements coalesce to create an environment that can restore a weary spirit.

Moreover, time spent in green spaces fosters a profound connection with the living world, nurturing our innate biophilia. As we align our fitness endeavours with the cadence of the natural world, we inadvertently begin to care more deeply for it. Environmental stewardship, then, may just evolve as an unexpected but cherished side-effect of our outdoor fitness pursuits.

Meditative practices are another treasure trove when set against the backdrop of greenery. Yoga on the grass, tai chi near the whispering reeds of a pond, or a mindfulness session within the protective circle of an arboreal amphitheatre—the synergy of these activities with nature can lead to profound moments of clarity and peace.

Let's not overlook the social dimension either. Green spaces are unique in their ability to foster community and shared experiences. Group workouts, boot camps, and family picnics within these natural settings can all contribute to the communal bond, amplifying the therapeutic effects through the joy of togetherness. In every shared laugh and cheer, we find an intangible medicine that no clinic could dispense.

Yet, despite these odes to nature's healing prowess, barriers persist. Time constraints, accessibility issues, or even personal discomfort with outdoor conditions can all dissuade individuals from benefitting from green spaces. It's our mission, then, to tear down these walls, to reimagine urban planning with health and wellness interwoven into its blueprint. Cities must not only accommodate but also encourage these natural sanctuaries for their residents' holistic health.

Envision a city where every neighbourhood basks in the embrace of its very own green haven. Here, the concrete jungle yields to verdant retreats, providing therapeutic environments accessible to all, regardless of socio-economic standing. This isn't just utopian dreaming but a public health strategy to enhance the quality of life for inhabitants spanning every corner of our urban landscapes.

In recognising the therapeutic value of green spaces, we must ensure their presence isn't relegated to the outskirts, available only to those with the leisure and means to reach them. Instead, a mosaic of mini-parks, green corridors, and community gardens should be interwoven into the fabric of our daily lives.

And let's not settle for mere space preservation. Active efforts towards nurturing and expanding these areas are crucial. Every planted tree, every restored wetland, and every protected meadow can become a potential haven for someone in need of nature's restorative touch. Such initiatives breathe life back not only into the environment but also into the communities they serve.

As our cities burgeon and technology tethers us ever tighter to screens and artificial constructs, the need for green spaces – as places of wellness, social cohesion, and simple beauty – has never been more pressing. In the grand tapestry of health, threads of green are essential weaves, without which the picture is incomplete.

Let us cherish and protect these verdant lifelines, and may we collectively strive to create a world where green spaces are not luxuries but staples – integrated fully into the lives and routines of all who seek balance, health, and harmony.

So, lace up your shoes—not to run from something, but towards a sanctuary of growth. Let each step be a commitment to intertwining our fitness journeys with nature's pathways. After all, it is in the heart of these green spaces that many find not just solace, but a profound reminder of their own vitality. It is there, amidst the symphony of the natural world, that we can all tune in to the fine balance of life— challenged, restored, and ever flourishing.

Nature's Role in Physical and Emotional Recovery

We've often heard it said that a walk in the park can do wonders for the soul. Still, recent studies and countless personal experiences are drilling down into precisely how nature supports recovery, not just as a comforting backdrop but as an active participant in our healing journeys. Whether we're mending a broken bone or a worn-out spirit, Mother Nature has a remedy at the ready.

Consider the role of fresh air and sunlight in bolstering our body's defenses. Sunlight is a natural source of vitamin D, and vitamin D is crucial for bone health and immune system function – both indispensable parts of physical recovery. But that's just skimming the surface. The full-spectrum light from the sun can uplift our mood, potentially easing symptoms of depression and anxiety that often accompany the convalescence period.

The soothing sights and sounds of the outdoors, as well, seem tailor-made to calm a frazzled nervous system. Picture this: you're sitting by a meandering river, gazing at the languid flow of clear water, listening to the gentle rustle of leaves – a sensory experience that beckons your body towards rest and regeneration. It's no accident that these stimuli can lower our blood pressure and slow our heart rate; they're nature's subtle signals that it's time for healing.

There's also the undeniable connection between natural landscapes and our mental well-being. Engaging in outdoor physical activities reduces symptoms of stress and anxiety. When we hit that forest trail or park path, cortisol levels – our body's stress hormones – begin to decrease. As the stress dissipates, our body can turn its efforts towards repair and renewal.

It is not just about the physical aspects, either. Emotional recovery often requires a mental reset – a chance to step away from our daily grind and the pollutants of a busy mind. When you immerse yourself into the wilderness, you're casting aside your usual stimuli for something more primal and grounding. In the absence of to-do lists and traffic, you find space to process events, which can be immensely healing.

Moving beyond the conventional, researchers are now exploring the concept of ecotherapy – where interaction with nature is prescribed to assist with mental health issues. The term may be recent, but the practice is as old as time. It's about reconnecting with the earth, with life's simple cycles, to remember our place in the larger schema of existence.

Nature's impact extends to helping us deal with grief and loss. A walk in the woods can be reflective, a way to step out of time, to feel the continuity of life – the growing tree, the constant babble of a brook – and to come to terms with our transient yet impactful spot in this continuum.

Furthermore, nature can be a catalyst for social healing. Outdoor group activities not only foster peer support but allow shared experiences to reinforce our sense of community and belonging. This social aspect can be significant for those who feel isolated due to trauma or illness, offering a bridge back to a world they may have felt disconnected from.

What about the tactile element? Gardening, for instance, offers a literal hands-on connection with the earth. This not just creates a sense of accomplishment and caretaking, but it also involves beneficial bacteria in the soil that may boost our serotonin levels – a natural antidepressant.

For the adventurers among us, nature challenges our physical limits, too. Rock climbing, for example, isn't just about the thrill; it's about reclaiming strength, testing our resilience, and overcoming limitations that we've come up against in our recovery process. It instills a sense of achievement that's both physically and psychologically restorative.

Healing spaces have also become a fundamental aspect of recuperative environments. Hospitals with rooms that offer views of greenery have reported improved outcomes for patients. It begs the question – if such passive interaction can make a difference, what can active engagement accomplish?

Water is another element that complements our healing. Hydrotherapy, long recognized for its therapeutic benefits, encompasses everything from a swim in the lake to the gentle rhythm of coastal waves helping to restore balance and promote inner tranquility.

Finally, we mustn't overlook the benefit of just pure silence that nature can provide. In our increasingly noisy world, the quietude of a snow-covered peak or a misty morning in a meadow grants us a reprieve from the clamour. Silence can be as restorative as sleep, giving our brains a much-needed break to recharge and recover.

In closing, whether you're patching up an injured limb or seeking solace for a weary heart, the therapeutic embrace of nature is readily available. It's an ally that constantly beckons us towards growth, resilience, and well-being. And in turning to the natural world for recovery, we're not just healing ourselves; we're forging a connection to something eternal and understanding our role within it all.

To sum up, nature's gym doesn't just condition our bodies; it can become a profound part of our healing. When we step outside and commune with the elements in their raw form, we're giving ourselves a chance to take part in something inexplicably powerful – the timeless cycle of rest, recovery, and rejuvenation that mother nature so effortlessly showcases.

Chapter 22:
The Nature's Gym Success Stories

Inspirational tales aren't just found in far-off legends; they're blossoming around us, rooted in the very soil we tread during our outdoor adventures. *The Nature's Gym Success Stories* is a patchwork quilt of personal triumphs and metamorphoses, all sewn together by the common thread of the great outdoors. Each narrative is a fresh flower in a meadow of motivation; from the office worker who traded his treadmill for mountain trails, redefining his limits with each summit conquered, to the stay-at-home parent who found community and strength through a local outdoor fitness tribe, and the retiree who discovered that her true vitality began at the edge of a lake at sunrise, with the discipline of her morning swims. The elements served as both obstacle and ally, forging not just physical robustness but a fortified spirit resilient against life's undulating challenges. These accounts do more than stir the spirit; they showcase the enduring power of outdoor fitness to sculpt a steadfast lifestyle, enhancing health and serenity through every season's turn.

Inspirational Accounts of Transformation

Outdoor endeavours often provide the backdrop for the most profound transformations. Imagine shedding the office constraints, the blaring city noise, and stepping into an adventure under the open sky, where every breath of fresh air whispers of potential.

Let me tell you about Mia. Mia's real-time transformation began with a simple stroll through a park, her sanctuary away from a high-stress tech job. But over time, the trails called her name, luring her toward verdant woodlands and mountainsides that demanded stamina and grit. What started as leisurely walks evolved into regular hikes, each one chiselling away at her stress, sculpting a more robust sense of self, until one day, she realised she had not just conquered miles but personal milestones too.

Then, there's James, already an athlete, but one accustomed to the gym's mirrored walls. It wasn't until a friend coaxed him out for a trail run that his perception of true fitness expanded. Nature's unremitting terrains reshaped his understanding of strength and endurance. James found his rhythm amidst the rustling leaves and babbling streams, his running shoes pounding a new beat, a beat that echoed the resilience he was building with every outdoor workout.

For Priya, transformation came on two wheels, mendling the rapture of riding with the thrill of unpredictable paths. The local cycling club introduced her to off-road biking, which swiftly shifted her focus from counting calories to mastering trails. The bike became an instrument of joy rather than an odometer of exertion, and this joy recharged her zest for life.

Consider the retirees, Sam and Anita, who traded long hours on the couch for birdwatching expeditions. Initially armed with binoculars for casual observation, their backyard hobby transcended to passionate treks through remote landscapes. Their stamina improved, their connection deepened—not just with nature, but with each other, reaffirming that transformation through nature's embrace knows no age.

Dan's story is about swapping the treadmill for the rugged coastlines. A journey from the mundane to the magnificent, as he describes it. The measured predictability of a conveyor belt beneath his feet paled in comparison to the rich tapestry of sandy shores, coastal flora, and the rolling sea. The salt air didn't just fill his lungs; it infused his life with a fresh sense of purpose and a briny zest you can't find in a gym.

Lucy's metamorphosis was through moving meditations in nature, where each mountaintop brought not just panoramic views, but clarity and peace of mind. Yoga by the riverbanks and tai chi in meadow clearings taught her that the stillness of the body in nature could lead to profound internal movement and growth.

For Carlos, adaptation meant acclimatizing to the chill of dawn runs. And as the seasons changed, so did he, transitioning from dreading the cold to appreciating the crisp clarity it brought to his morning rituals. This new-found fervour for the chillier hours paved the way for Carlos to test his warmth in winter sports, further pushing the boundaries of his comfort zone.

Not all stories embody dramatic life changes; take Rachel, who integrated lunchtime walks into her daily routine. These intermissions amidst greenery reinvigorated her workday, boosting productivity and creativity. It was a subtle yet significant shift, illustrating that even minor edits in our daily manuscript can lead to chapters of well-being.

Equally compelling are tales of recovery, like Mark's. Following a cycling accident, the outdoors became both his respite and his rehab centre. Physical therapy sessions extended into the park, where each step forward was a breath of hope, a stretch toward his former vitality. Mother Nature's restorative powers played a pivotal role in his healing, both physical and emotional.

What's common to these narratives is the staging ground – the great outdoors. It's where challenges are accepted, limits are pushed, and transformations occur not in huge revelations, but through the compounding effect of daily choices and consistent efforts. It's where life's tumult gives way to trails and tribulation becomes triumph.

Surely, the myriad of equipment we surround ourselves can't compare with the organic, raw gym that nature provides, where every tool for transformation is alive, dynamic, and often, therapeutic. The open-air gym doesn't come with monthly fees; rather it pays dividends in health, happiness, and harmony with the earth.

Each of these inspirational transformations stands as testament to nature's gym's versatility and it's vital not to forget that it is accessible to all. Whether you're embarking on a personal challenge or are a seasoned outdoor enthusiast, the call of the wild is inclusive, inviting you to carve out your own path of transformation.

It's not confined by walls or limited to urban parks. The raw beauty of remote landscapes is equally transformative. As we'll explore in later chapters, immersing oneself in the untouched wild can amplify the senses, redefine perspectives and renew our appreciation for the planet's magnificence.

And so, these stories are here to ignite a spark, to reinforce that outdoor activity is a catalyst for change. They are beacons lighting the way, illuminating paths that others have trodden in their pursuit of wellness through every changing season. Stories that resonate with progress made amidst the sun, rain, wind, and snow—stories that inspire you to take that step outside and witness your own transformation in nature's ever-present gym.

The Long-Term Benefits of Outdoor Fitness

As we dive deeper into the journey of fitness and well-being, there's a sanctuary we often overlook—the great outdoors. Imagine the open sky as your ceiling and the earth beneath your feet, a limitless territory to explore and engage your entire being.

Outdoor fitness isn't just another avenue to burn calories or achieve a summer body. It's a pathway to profound wellness, one that intertwines with the threads of nature to create a tapestry of enduring health benefits. The landscape of outdoor fitness is rich and varied, much like the seasons themselves.

The benefits of outdoor fitness unfold gradually, and over time they compile a list longer than the trails you'll tread. Beyond the immediate rush of endorphins and the satisfaction of a workout well done, there's a deeper connection taking root. Let's peel back the layers and discover the lasting gifts that nature bestows on those who engage regularly in outdoor training.

One of the most significant long-term benefits is the influence of outdoor fitness on mental health. It's clear that regular exposure to natural environments can sharpen the mind and lighten the mood. The serenity of a park, the whimsical dance of a leaf, and the fragrance of a forest after rain, all contribute to alleviating anxiety and combatting depression.

Cardiovascular health is another major beneficiary of consistent outdoor activity. Cycling up a hill, running along a trail, or even a brisk walk in the park can help reduce the risk of heart disease. It's the gift that keeps on giving; with each beat of your heart, you're pumping towards a stronger, more resilient you.

In relation to skeletal strength and integrity, the terrain of the outdoors offers resistance and variation that a flat treadmill simply cannot compete with. Commanding your body to navigate uneven grounds translates to improved bone density and a fortified skeletal system, guarding against the ravages of osteoporosis in later life.

Outdoor fitness is also a silent warrior in the fight against chronic conditions. Whether it's maintaining insulin sensitivity to combat diabetes or improving circulation to keep blood pressure in check, the dance with nature can be a preventive melody for many health concerns.

Vitamin D, the sunshine vitamin, is often in scant supply, especially in indoor-focused lifestyles. Regular outdoor activity ensures your body can naturally procure this essential nutrient, fostering better immune function and bone health. It's the body's way of thanking you for stepping out under the sky's vast canvas.

The sensory engagement that comes from working out amidst flora and fauna is unmatched. The scent of pine, the sound of a stream, the feel of the breeze against your skin—all these elements combine to enhance your workout experience, anchoring you firmly in the present moment, a form of physical mindfulness in action.

In terms of weight management, the diversity of outdoor environments encourages the body to adapt continuously, often leading to more calories burned over time compared to indoor exercises. Those who find their gym within nature's walls tend to stick with their routines longer, fostering a lifelong relationship with fitness.

Another long-term advantage is the versatility that outdoor fitness offers. Nature's gym is open to all, regardless of income or social status. This democratic approach to exercise embraces inclusivity, allowing more people to reap the long-term rewards of a fit and active lifestyle.

Outdoor fitness also has a knack for nurturing social connections. Joining a hiking group or pairing up with a jogging buddy, it forms communities—networks of support that enhance the social aspect of wellbeing. It's been shown that such support can lead to greater consistency and longevity in maintaining an active lifestyle.

The environmental aspect of outdoor fitness is often underappreciated. It's a gentle reminder of our role as stewards of the planet. As you benefit from nature, you tend to develop an innate desire to protect it, nurturing a long-term commitment to environmental conservation and sustainability.

Beyond the physical and mental upshots, outdoor fitness imparts a sense of adventure and curiosity. It's an invitation to expand horizons, to discover hidden paths and trails. This exploratory spirit enriches life, keeps the sense of wonder alive and can remain well into the golden years of life.

Lastly, but by no means least, the spiritual enrichment that comes with regular communion with nature cannot be overlooked. For many, the great outdoors is a sacred space, providing solace and introspection. It is in these moments of solitude that one often finds clarity and a renewed sense of purpose.

Wrapping up, the long-term benefits of outdoor fitness span the spectrum of human health and experience. They build a foundation that is robust and resilient, capable of weathering life's storms. It's a holistic investment, where the dividends pay out in physical vitality, mental clarity, social connectedness, environmental responsibility, and spiritual fulfilment. Embrace outdoor fitness not just as a transient trend, but as a lifelong ally in the quest for comprehensive well-being.

Chapter 23:
The Environmental Footprint of Fitness

As we lace up our running shoes or gear up for a trek, it's crucial we pause and ponder the impact our fitness routine has on the very environment we cherish. Each sprint through the park, each paddle across the lake, we're not just building stamina but also leaving an imprint on nature's delicate canvas. Sustainable exercise isn't just a buzzword; it's a partnership with the planet that demands mindfulness. We've already embraced nature's gym, drawn to the whispering trees and rugged trails, and now we must protect it. This isn't merely about reducing plastic bottles by investing in a sturdy water flask, or choosing to bike rather than drive to our favourite outdoor spots—we need to consider the entire lifecycle of our gear, the erosion our footsteps might cause, and the wildlife whose homes we jog past. It's about finding that synergy between getting in shape and keeping the Earth fit, exploring eco-friendly fitness options and embracing responsible recreation practices. We've got the opportunity to turn every lung-busting hill climb into a statement of our respect for Mother Nature, one where we do not merely take from but give back and ensure the continuity of this wondrous outdoor gymnasium. Our fitness journey is intertwined with the environment's wellbeing—let's make every step count towards preserving nature's beauty.

Responsible Recreation: Preserving Nature's Beauty

Following our pursuit of year-round fitness in the throes of nature's bounty, it's essential to consider the impact we leave behind where tread meets trail. Just as seasons evoke transformation across landscapes, our interactions with the environment should reflect a responsible stewardship. Immersing oneself in the outdoors endows a privilege that comes with a duty: to preserve the very spaces that afford us physical and mental rejuvenation.

So, let's take a moment to navigate the ethos of 'leave no trace' which underpins responsible recreation. Keen as we are to chase horizons and conquer peaks, our forays into the green should be marked by an invisible presence, allowing nature's orchestra to play unabridged, uninterrupted by our footprints. This entails sticking to established trails, which serve to concentrate foot traffic and limit soil erosion and vegetation loss.

As outdoor aficionados, we must kindle a symbiotic relationship with our surroundings. This means setting up camps, when embraced by nature's canopy, on durable surfaces. The principle is simple: use areas that are resilient to wear. By doing so, we honour the pact made with the earth to cause minimal scarring on its visage.

Equally paramount is the practice of disposing of waste properly. One might think an apple core or handful of nuts being biodegradable means they can be gifted back to the earth. However, these leftovers are foreign to the ecosystems and could be detrimental to local fauna. Pack it in, pack it out – this mantra should echo within our minds, ensuring all our rubbish returns with us, leaving behind nothing but the rustle of leaves.

It's not simply what we leave behind that counts, but also what we don't take. Flowers, rocks and natural artefacts are visual sonnets, each telling a tale of their native residence. To uproot, pocket or carry these away is to rob the landscape of its voice. Photographs and memories are the true souvenirs we should harvest from our excursions.

Sound also carries weight in the outdoor arena. Our vocal emissions should be measured, an effort to respect the audial landscape and other adventurers seeking solace in nature's quietude. Conversations and exclamations should not compete with the whispers of leaves and the chatter of wildlife. Soft words foster the inclusive enjoyment and sanctuary of open space.

Engaging with wildlife should be a distant admiration—a theatre of life observed from the back row. Feeding animals or encroaching for a closer look disrupts their inherent behaviour patterns and could potentially endanger both parties. Let's remember that we are guests in their home, and as such, our conduct should reflect a courteous visitor.

Consider fires within nature's gym. While the dance of flames might allure, know that many ecosystems are susceptible to the scars of fire. Use stoves for cooking, and where open flames are permitted, ensure they're kept small, managed responsibly, and thoroughly extinguished. Ashes and remnants should be as ephemeral as the warmth enjoyed.

Hiking and camping gear should also be environmentally considerate. Products free from harsh chemicals, biodegradable soaps, and renewable materials are just some of the ways equipment choices can reflect our eco-commitment. Let's scrutinise our purchases through the lens of sustainability, picking brands and items that champion eco-friendly practices.

Companionship on the trail goes beyond human cohorts to include the four-legged kind. Responsible pet ownership means acknowledging certain spaces may impose restrictions on our furry friends. Where they are welcome, ensure they are under control, for the safety of wildlife, the environment, and other recreators immersed in their journey.

When nature narrates its gusto through weather—may it be the gale's howl or the rain's rhythm—respect her dialogue. Storms carve and shape the encompassing canvas. Risking our safety or the integrity of the terrain because we've defied weather warnings does a disservice to the ethos of outdoor stewardship.

Responsible recreation entails educating ourselves and others. Knowledge is the torchlight that can illuminate the path to environmental preservation. Whether it's a novice hiker or a seasoned climber, each narrative enriched with ecological consideration strengthens the communal resolve to safeguard our natural theatres.

It's also about planning and preparation. Anticipate the demands of your outdoor excursions and assess the fragility of the ecosystems you'll explore. This forethought reduces the chances of unwelcome surprises that could lead to environmental degradation.

Vernal pools, summer meadows, autumn forests, and winter's white—each season presents a unique set of considerations for nature's gym users. Adjust your practices and equipment accordingly. The delicate blooms of spring require a lighter step, while the dormant landscapes of winter a sterner regard for the hidden life beneath the snow.

In closing, the pursuit of health through nature's varied gymnasium must be married with an ethos of preservation. Each droplet of sweat shed, each breath deepened by exertion, binds us more closely to the natural world and its rhythmic cycles. Let us reciprocate with thoughtful action—to preserve, to protect, and to pass on nature's beauty unspoiled for generations that follow in our trail-blazing wake, seeking what we have found and cherished.

Sustainable Exercise: Eco-Friendly Fitness Options

Embarking on a journey of physical well-being can also be a commitment to the health of our planet. Our strides, our swims, and even our cycles resonate with more than personal gains—they touch the earth itself. Let's explore how our fitness can tread lightly, leaving a faint footprint behind, supported by the very soil we so often take for granted in our pursuit of wellness.

The conversation about eco-friendly fitness often starts with the mode of activity. Running, an activity with minimal equipment, naturally springs to mind. Yet there's room to take it further. Have you considered the production and disposal impact of your running shoes, or sought out brands that advocate for sustainability in their materials and processes? It's a step that aligns your gym with the greenery around you.

The beauty of pedal power can't be overstated—bicycling for fitness isn't just about toned calves and a robust cardio workout. It's a vehicle for change, often literally. Sustainable exercise includes using bikes made from recycled materials, engaging in pedal-powered community events, and championing local infrastructure that supports bike-based commuting.

Indeed, water-based exercises hold their own in environmental stewardship. Open water swimming, kayaking, and paddleboarding all harness natural elements for fitness, free from the confining swim lanes of chlorine-filled pools. The call is not only to dive in but to contribute to maintaining our waterways' cleanliness—participating in waterborne litter collections merges an upper-body workout with aquatic conservation efforts.

Adopting a mindful approach to location is vital in eco-friendly fitness. The concept is simple: opt for natural spaces within walking or cycling distance. If you must drive, how about shared transportation to the trailhead? Moreover, this proximity encourages regular engagement with your outdoor gym, folding exercise into your daily life seamlessly.

Then there's the matter of energy consumption. Off-grid workouts that shun electronic devices and machines, instead using one's own body weight or the resistance provided by nature, epitomise sustainable exercise. Think calisthenics in the park, hill sprints, or even utilising fallen branches or rocks for strength training—nature is abundant with equipment if we only choose to see it.

The shift to an eco-conscious workout routine also invites an assessment of workout wear. Choosing attire made from sustainable, organic, or recycled materials complements your routines with respect for the resources used. Furthermore, durability in these items means less waste, fewer items purchased over time, and a kind of timeless fashion that withstands fleeting trends.

Practices such as foraging during hikes or runs transform exercise into a symbiotic relationship with the land. Gathering wild berries or herbs not only educates on local flora but also promotes a diet rooted in the seasonal and regional, reducing reliance on transported goods— a small step towards mitigating your meals' carbon footprint.

But it's not just the 'what' or 'where' that forms the backbone of sustainable exercise—it's also the 'how'. Sticking to marked trails, for instance, protects vulnerable ecosystems from erosion or damage and keeps wild habitats undisturbed, demonstrating a balance between fitness activity and ecological preservation.

Group fitness activities also offer an opportunity for communal environmental responsibility. Whether it's a low-impact yoga session in a serene glade or a team sport on the beach using a reusable net, social workouts can emphasise resourcefulness and shared environmental ethics. Collective transport to these events further reduces the ecological impact.

The seasonality of certain activities inherently embraces eco-friendliness. Snowshoeing in winter or surfing in summer uses the seasonal environment to its advantage, requiring little more than the correct conditions provided by mother nature herself. By adapting to the seasons, we yield to nature's rhythm and accept her invitation to fitness with minimal environmental disturbance.

Urban dwellers aren't excluded from this green fitness revolution. Substituting gym time with park workouts, stair climbing, or engaging in community gardening are all ways to maintain fitness levels while contributing to the environmental wealth of urban settings. What's more is that these practices often lead to the development of green corridors within cities, which foster biodiversity and provide a breath of fresh air—quite literally.

Of course, there are occasions when indoor training is preferable or necessary. In such moments, the sustainable mindset needn't be abandoned. Choosing eco-friendly equipment within gyms, or leveraging natural light and ventilation, ensures that even when sheltered from the elements, our environment remains a forethought. Therefore, when the storm clouds gather, and the outdoors isn't an option, the commitment to eco-friendly fitness stands firm.

Lastly, digital tools and apps can help track the environmental impact of workouts. They can suggest the most eco-friendly routes, help to locate outdoor exercise groups nearby or even provide guidance on reducing waste while staying active. In a world where technology can be a drain on resources, this is one way it can contribute positively to our ecological fitness footprint.

By weaving sustainability into the fabric of our fitness lives, we don't just benefit our bodies; we nourish the very earth that enables us.

It's a powerful exchange, a dialogue between individual health and the wellbeing of our planet. So, let's pull on sustainably made trainers, swim in clean lakes, bike on recycled wheels, and forge a path forward where every step, every stroke, and every pedal is a testament to a thriving, symbiotic existence with our environment.

Chapter 24:
Weathering the Storm:
When Outdoor Isn't an Option

There are days when the skies turn sombre and the raging tempests render our beloved outdoor gym inaccessible. But don't you think for a second that's a reason to throw in the towel. We've all felt that pang of disappointment when lacing up our trainers only to come face-to-face with a torrential downpour or an unforgiving blizzard. Yet, this is precisely the moment to tap into a well of creativity and resilience that nature herself teaches us. Within the four walls of our homes, we can conjure up a sanctuary that mirrors the tranquility and challenge of the outdoors. By bringing elements of nature inside, like potted plants that oxygenate your space or playing a soundscape of rustling leaves and chirping birds, your indoor environment transforms into a makeshift haven of natural harmony. Guidance on crafting your domestic nature-nook will be in the coming pages, along with strategies to maintain peak fitness when extreme weather slams the door shut on outdoor activities. So hang tight, because the storm doesn't pause our pursuit—it simply adds a twist to the trail.

Creating an Indoor Nature Experience

Imagine it's one of those days when the weather isn't cooperating, or perhaps you're pinned down by a bout of stormy forecasts. Rather than feeling cooped up and disconnected from the rejuvenating pulse of the outdoors, there's a spectrum of ways to infuse your indoor space with the essence of the natural world. Creating an indoor nature experience isn't just about aesthetics; it's about engagement, interaction, and invoking a sense of place that mirrors the great outdoors.

Start with light. If you've ever lingered in a beam of sunlight streaming through a window, you'll know the warmth and comfort it can bring. It's about recreating those conditions as best you can. Whether that's repositioning furniture to be bathed in natural light or choosing full-spectrum light bulbs that mimic daylight, these subtle changes can prompt your body into the rhythm of the outdoors, even when you're inside.

Then there are plants – an indoor jungle can turn a stagnant room into a living space. It's not just their vibrant green hues that ignite a sense of vitality but also their ability to purify the air, turning your home into a fresh, oxygen-rich environment. From spider plants to peace lilies, choose varieties that thrive indoors and require a level of care that fits your routine.

But a visual connection to nature isn't enough; your other senses need to be catered to as well. Consider a small indoor water feature – the sound of trickling water can transport you to a serene mountain stream or a gentle rain shower. It has a calming effect, reminiscent of stepping outside after the rain and hearing the droplets fall from leaves.

The tactility of nature can be echoed through materials and textures too. Stone, wood, and natural fibres can be included in your decor to simulate the touch of the outdoors. A bamboo mat or a chunk of pine wood can become keystones of your indoor nature sanctuary. Walk over them barefoot, and you're traipsing through the landscape in the comfort of your own home.

Aromas play an intrinsic role in how we perceive our environment. Pine-scented candles, eucalyptus sprays, or simply opening the windows to let in fresh air can revitalize your indoor experience. These scent notes can have profound effects on mood and memory, serving as an invisible thread tying you to the outdoor realms.

We can't overlook the soundscapes of nature either. Ambient recordings of forest sounds, ocean waves, or birdsong, played quietly in the background, can fill the absence of natural noise pollution in our homes. These audio cues don't just inject a natural soundtrack into your space – they can have soothing effects on your psyche, much like the real thing.

Next up, incorporating earthy colours into your interior design can evoke the palette of the outdoors. Whether that's through cushions, wall paint, or artwork, surrounding yourself with colours you might find on a mountain trail or a beachscape sustains the connection with nature. It's about replicating the hues that stir your soul when you're out in the wild.

You might also explore terrariums as a microcosm of the natural world. Building a tiny ecosystem within a glass container is not just a soothing hobby; it's a concentrated dose of nature that you can marvel at from your desk or coffee table. These miniature landscapes require observation and engagement, helping you stay attuned to the subtleties of natural life.

Incorporating natural elements into your workout space can be transformative as well. A room dedicated to indoor fitness becomes even more inviting when complemented by natural elements. A sand-filled Zen garden to meditate next to after a workout, or weights made from natural materials, can reinforce the idea that you're training in nature's gym, regardless of your locale.

Virtual reality can offer an escape into natural worlds beyond our immediate reach. Immersive programs can simulate treks through virtual forests or mountaintops, providing sensorial depictions of the outdoors that can inspire and energise. This technology, though artificial, taps into our innate desire to roam freely and explore.

Eating fresh, whole foods as you would during outdoor activities is part of experiencing nature indoors. Serve up a platter of seasonal produce, perhaps from your local farmer's market or even your own windowsill garden, and you're not just nourishing your body; you're living a lifestyle congruent with your desire for a connection with nature.

Interactive elements such as wildlife webcams or live feeds from national parks can create dynamic windows into environments far from your home. With technology enabling real-time connections to different parts of the globe, you might catch a glimpse of a bear in North America or a tropical thunderstorm in real-time, expanding your indoor nature experience globally.

Finally, in crafting your indoor nature experience, don't forget the influence of art. Photographs, paintings, or sculptures that reflect the natural world can act as daily reminders of where you'd rather be. They are silent motivators, bolstering your spirit until you can next step outside and embrace the elements again.

Adapting to the ebb and flow of life's circumstances, including weather extremes, doesn't mean we should sever our ties with nature. On the contrary, it's about seizing the opportunity to be innovative and immersive in cultivating a nature experience within our four walls. Doing so helps maintain that essential connection that nurtures our minds, bodies, and souls.

So, as we consider the enchantment that the outdoors holds for our overall well-being, let this be a testament to our incredible human capacity to adapt and thrive. By creating an indoor nature experience, we pay homage to the outdoors, reiterating its importance in our daily lives and ensuring that our connection to nature remains vibrant, even when we've temporarily retreated indoors.

Staying Fit During Extreme Weather

As dedicated pursuers of outdoor adventures, sometimes we're challenged by Mother Nature's less forgiving moods. Blistering heatwaves, bone-chilling cold snaps, and unforeseen storms can turn a routine fitness endeavour into a test of wills. But let's not be daunted! Instead, let's see these occasions as opportunities to adapt, improvise, and overcome – ensuring our fitness journey is uninterrupted, regardless of the skies above.

First off, let's tackle the sweltering heat that can besiege our summers. High temperatures needn't scorch our exercise routines if we're smart about it. The early bird catches the cooler morning – or the evening owl enjoys the night's reprieve. Timing workouts to avoid peak heat isn't just about comfort; it's about safety as well. Don't forget to cloak your skin with sweat-proof sunscreen and dress in breathable fabrics that wick away perspiration.

Hydration, as we're all aware, is a cornerstone of exercise, more so during heat waves. Ensuring you have a reliable source of water while you workout isn't negotiable. And while we're on essentials, let's not forget that replenishing salts and minerals with an electrolyte-infused drink can be a game-changer when pushing through heat barriers.

Flipping the thermostat now, let's pivot to the icy edges of the spectrum. When winter wields its frosty hand, layering intelligently is your armour against the cold. Merino wools and synthetics should sit close to your skin, trapping warmth while steering clear of cotton that loves to hold damp like a sponge. Remember, the aim is to stay warm without overheating or becoming a sponge for sweat.

As the sleet pounds the pavements, the lure of indoor workouts can tug insistently. But have you ever felt the invigorating zap of cold air as you jog through a silent park, snowflakes conspiring to turn the world into a monochrome masterpiece? That feeling is irreplaceable. It's the blend of adrenaline and endorphins – a winter's cocktail served fresh by the great outdoors.

Should a blizzard blow through, however, common sense dictates we find alternatives. Bodyweight regimes, yoga flows, or a high-energy dance workout at home can keep the metabolic fires burning. Preparation for such inevitabilities means having a home-based workout routine in your arsenal, so that a snowy day doesn't become a no-gym day.

Now, what about those sudden deluges or relentless downpours? Rain needn't be a deterrent. It can be quite the ally, with the rhythmic patter setting a steady pace for your runs. Just don a waterproof jacket, secure your electronics, and choose a path less likely to pool with water. Trust me, there's a unique joy in returning home, drenched on the surface but dry and toasty underneath.

Heart-pounding windstorms might make you think twice about heading out. But they can also provide natural resistance training. Cycling or running into the wind builds stamina and strength – it's the earth's very own resistance band. If you're concerned about being blown off course, stick to routes with natural windbreakers like buildings, trees, or hills.

Wildfires, while rarer, do pose significant risks, especially with air quality. When the air turns acrid with smoke, indoor exercise is the responsible choice. Air filters and staying hydrated can help mitigate the risks of indoor pollutants, keeping your lungs as clear as possible while the world outside recovers.

Extreme weather can also deliver surges of humidity that turn the air thick as soup. Cooling vests, staying in the shade, and utilising moisture-absorbing powders can make a muggy day bearable. Adjusting intensity on these steamy sessions is wise, so go for consistent, lower-impact exercises to maintain stamina without overheating.

During those sombre times when the weather warning signs flash red, and authorities advise against venturing out, let's take it seriously. The beauty of fitness today is its versatility. Circuits, online workout classes, stair climbing, or even corridor sprints – you can keep your body moving within the protection of your abode. You'd be surprised at just how creative one can get with household items and a pinch of imagination.

Speaking of creativity, maybe this is the perfect moment to explore new realms of fitness. Yoga, Pilates, or Tai Chi can offer serenity amidst the storm, helping you cultivate calm within the chaos. These practices not only train the body but the mind as well, reinforcing the mental fortitude we need to face nature's more extreme moments.

Extreme weather doesn't just test our physical readiness; it's a mirror reflecting our preparation mindset. It asks us to consider all possible scenarios and equip ourselves with knowledge, backup plans, and the right gear. It's the sure-footedness that comes from knowing today's storm is just tomorrow's training anecdote.

Mind, let's not play light with our wellbeing. Regularly check forecasts, understand what your environment is capable of, and know when to hold back. It's not conceding defeat; it's picking your battles wisely, ensuring you're ready to seize the next clear day with gusto.

Ultimately, our engagement with nature's unpredictability sharpens our resilience and grit. Let's not forget, fitness is a decision – a commitment that doesn't get weathered down by storms or sunbeams. Every drop of rain, every snowflake, each gust of wind is an invitation, not an impedance. So don your layers, gear up, hydrate, and arm yourself with a plan. The great outdoors, in all its temperamental glory, awaits.

Chapter 25:
The Future of Outdoor Fitness

As we peer over the horizon, it's vividly clear that the trajectory of outdoor fitness is aligning more and more with cutting-edge technology, innovatively weaving together the innate human desire for natural spaces with the digital age's conveniences. Imagine a time where bio-sensing wearables don't just track our vitals but also suggest real-time route changes to enhance our workouts with the ideal balance of sun, shade, and terrain. Drones could become our new jogging companions, capturing our progress while offering aerial cues and encouragement. Yet, amidst this rush towards tech integration, it's the timeless call of the raw, untamed wilderness that consistently lures us out of our high-tech cocoons, reminding us that the touch of the earth beneath our feet and the rhythm of the seasons can't be synthesized. As we embrace the unparalleled potential that the future holds, let's champion an evolution of outdoor fitness that not only sophisticates our experience but also deepens our connection to the pulse of the planet. After all, it's this synergy between advancement and the ancient cadence of nature that will sculpt the next chapter of our journey towards holistic well-being.

Technological Advances and Nature's Gym

The lines between technology and our interaction with the natural world are blurring. Picture this: You're on a run through the woods, the only sounds are your footsteps and the forest around you. Yet, on your wrist, a smartwatch buzzes with real-time data on your heart rate, distance covered, and elevation climbed. Step by step, we're discovering that technology doesn't have to pull us away from nature—it can actually enhance our connection with the outdoors.

Consider the GPS devices that have revolutionised trekking. Their sophisticated systems don't merely show you a dot on a map but provide high-resolution 3D terrain views, allowing for safe explorations into previously intimidating landscapes. Scrolling through waypoints isn't just practical; it's a way to invite certainty into the embrace of the unpredictable wild.

Now, let's talk about wearable tech. These nifty little devices track our exertions, sleep, and even suggest recovery times. Sure, a bit of gear will never replace the thrill of reaching a summit, but it can ensure you're fit enough to enjoy the ascent safely. It's like having a personal trainer strapped to your wrist, one who appreciates the value of fresh air and a good, rugged hill.

Advancements in material science are even transforming what we wear. Waterproof, breathable fabrics and ergonomically designed footwear allow for prolonged sojourns into nature's gym regardless of the weather. You might find yourself dancing in the rain rather than ducking for cover, thanks to gear that keeps you comfortably dry.

The rise of fitness apps and platforms that cater to outdoor enthusiasts is nothing short of a digital age boon. Virtual challenges entice us with badges and rewards for completing real-world hiking trails or marathon runs. It's gaming meets gains, and it's a fantastic way to stay motivated when the call of your couch feels a bit too tempting.

And then there are environmental sensors, small, hand-held devices or even smartphone attachments which allow the user to gain insights into the local air quality, temperature, humidity, and more. This sort of information can be a boon for those training at different altitudes or wanting to acclimatize to more challenging conditions gradually.

But technology doesn't only lend a hand in the actual doing. It's also transforming the planning. Digital maps, intricately detailed and updated in real time, feed the wanderlust of the modern adventurer. They plot the course for your next run, cycle, or open-water swim in granular, zoomable glory. You can curate an outing that tests your limits or one that soothes your soul, all from a device that fits in the palm of your hand.

Let's not gloss over the safety boost technology has provided. Emergency locator beacons and satellite communicators keep you connected even when you're off-grid, patiently waiting in your pack, offering peace of mind that help isn't as far away as you might think.

In the constant push and pull of engaging with the natural world, tech needn't be seen as an adversary. Our smartphones, if used mindfully, capture the glory of a mountain vista or the tranquil beauty of a hidden glen, ready to be shared or revisited during less adventurous days.

Even training aids, like suspension trainers or portable workout systems, have become more lightweight and nature-friendly. They allow for strength training by leveraging your own body weight, using nothing more than a sturdy tree branch as an anchor. It's an example of a workout that is simple in its essence but made versatile by intelligent design.

Augmented reality is another frontier where the natural and digital worlds collide. Imagine pointing your phone's camera at a plant and having an app instantly identify the species and its uses, or navigating a historical trail while overlaid stories and facts pop up to deepen the experience. This technology invites us to look at our environments with renewed curiosity and wonder.

Even in the realms of mental wellbeing, apps break down complex meditation and mindfulness techniques into prompts that guide us in real time, helping to find clarity and calm in the forests or mountains that surround us. It's inner peace crafted with an assist from the digital world.

As for the future, it's gleaming with even more integrated tech. Smart textiles promise clothing that can adapt to temperature changes or monitor muscle activation, providing data that pushes our understanding of human performance under nature's tutelage.

To wrap it up, technology in nature's gym is all about balance. By wielding the right tools with respect and understanding, we don't detract from the wild; we bring ourselves closer to it. We embrace a partnership with the outdoors that is informed, safe, and invigorating, ensuring that the footprint we leave on the earth is as gentle as the impact that the outdoors imprints on us.

Including another layer to our nature escapades doesn't mean we become less engaged with the environment. If anything, we become better listeners, more aware participants in the grand dialogue between human and earth. So next time you lace up your boots, consider how technology might not just shape your adventure, but enhance it in ways the explorers of yore could only have dreamt of.

Global Trends in Outdoor Activities and Fitness

The world is in constant motion, and the trends in outdoor activities and fitness are no exception. An invigorating synergy builds as the global community increasingly embraces the outdoors as the perfect playground for health and mindfulness. Let's cast a panoramic view over emerging trends that dovetail seamlessly with the indomitable spirit of adventure and the yearning for vitality.

Firstly, we're seeing a remarkable shift towards functional fitness regimes that mimic real-life activities — think rocking climbing, trail running, and parkour, weaving through grand cityscapes or natural terrains. These aren't just workouts; they're skills training sessions, where stamina and agility meet practicality and exhilaration. This shift invites a broader demographic to find their fit in outdoor activities, cultivating a refined appreciation for our innate physical capabilities.

Moreover, community-based fitness events, ranging from mud runs to obstacle course races, are seeing an upswing. These events foster a spirit of camaraderie and collective triumph over individual challenge. They often occur in spectacular settings, merging the appeal of raw natural beauty with the raw adrenaline of competition and shared experience.

The digital sphere intertwines with the physical through the growing popularity of fitness apps and wearable technology. These tools are revolutionizing how outdoor enthusiasts interact with their environment. From GPS tracking to monitor progress across mountain ridges, to apps that suggest hiking trails based on fitness levels, technology is an ever-present guide and motivator.

Sustainable travel has carved a niche in the fitness world with a strong push towards 'fitcations' — vacations designed around physical activities. This concept not only boosts local economies but also promotes environmental awareness and conservation as individuals engage with landscapes on a profound level.

Another development in global fitness is the increasing emphasis on low-impact activities, such as yoga and tai chi, held in outdoor settings. These mindful practices preach the harmony of movement, breath, and nature, attracting those who seek a holistic approach to well-being. Photographed against backdrops of serene lakes and sunrise-drenched mountains, these sessions are as much a feast for the eyes as they are nourishment for the body and soul.

In the realm of cycling, there's been a surge in gravel biking — it's the freedom of road cycling meets the grit of mountain biking. It embodies a desire for off-the-grid exploration, challenging oneself against the vagaries of untamed trails while embracing a more communal, less competitive cycling culture.

Water sports, too, are riding a new wave of interest. With stand-up paddleboarding, kayaking, and open-water swimming, there's something for everyone, from the tranquil paddler to the intrepid mariner. Each stroke under the open sky is a moment of connection with the very essence of our planet.

The inclusivity of outdoor fitness is expanding with movements that cater to those traditionally left out of the narrative. Adaptive sports programs throw open the gates of adventure to individuals with disabilities, championing the belief that the great outdoors is an arena for all.

Returning to the trails, there's a revival of interest in slow tourism. Hiking and walking holidays are cherished for their pace, which allows for deep immersion into the environment. It's not just about the physical exertion but also about the cultural exchange and the contemplative aspect of travel on foot.

Veganism and plant-based diets have made their way into the fitness trekker's backpack. The food fueling our expeditions mirrors a growing responsibility towards sustainability, compassion, and health. Foods once considered mere trail snacks are now key components of a conscious adventurer's diet.

Lastly, there's amplified importance being placed on 'leave no trace' principles and ecological responsibility. Today's fitness enthusiasts are tomorrow's stewards of the earth, striving to ensure their outdoor playground remains unspoiled for generations to come.

As we look towards the future, these trends paint a picture of a world where outdoor activities and fitness are bound by a common thread — the pursuit of a life well-lived, in harmony with our surroundings, with a touch of sustainable practice. Every step taken outside is an act of participation in a global movement toward better health, shared experiences, and environmental mindfulness.

In sum, the wave of outdoor fitness enthusiasts is as diverse as the landscapes they traverse. They are united by a quest for personal development and a commitment to preserving the natural world. Reflect on these trends as you lace up your shoes, secure your helmet, or take that first energizing breath of fresh air. The great outdoors awaits, not just as a backdrop for our fitness endeavors, but as a dynamic part of our collective journey to well-being.

In the chapters that follow, each season reveals unique opportunities and challenges, urging us to tailor our approach to stay aligned with these global trends in outdoor activities and fitness. Stay tuned, as we dive deeply into the toolkit of nature, harnessing its essence to foster a healthier, happier you.

Chapter 26:
The Year-Round Call of the Wild

As we close the pages of this enlightening journey through each chapter, filled with the vibrant heartbeat of nature's gym, let's take a moment to reflect. The great outdoors beckons us, irrespective of the season, offering a limitless playground for us to engage our minds and bodies in a symphony with the elements. Every season unfolds with its own unique call to the wild, a siren song that entices us to step beyond the familiar thresholds of our homes and into the vast expanse of nature.

The bracing air of spring reawakens our dormant senses, galvanising our spirits to set new intentions and pursue growth in tandem with the blossoming world around us. Then comes the fiery vitality of summer, daring us to push our physical limits under the watchful eye of the golden sun. Yet, it's not only about vigor and exposure; it's about finding balance in the fervor, learning to respect and adapt to the heat that both fuels and challenges us.

Autumn whispers the promise of transformation, nudging us to adapt our routines amidst the kaleidoscope of falling leaves. Here, we learn to embrace change not as a foe but as a friend, harmonising our movements with the crisp coolness that preludes the arrival of frosty days.

Winter then cloaks the landscape in a serene blanket of white, a wonderland that tempts the resilient. It's this season that often becomes the true test of our mettle. Building mental toughness, we learn that the right layers, along with indomitable spirit, can convert the chill into a crucible for fortitude and joy.

Inevitably, wet weather seeks to test our resolve. And yet, we find joy in dancing through the rain, our spirits unhampered by the whims of the clouds. Similarly, the wind, once seen as an adversary, becomes a dynamic partner in our outdoor enterprises, providing us with a fresh kind of resistance and balance to contend with.

The snow and ice are not merely obstacles; they present new arenas for play and practice, a crystalline challenge that teaches us poise and resilience, beckoning us to master the art of movement in the most slippery of circumstances.

Throughout each seasonal shift, we've explored the vital role of equipment – the physical extensions of our commitment to the wild. This gear, both a shield and a tool, has facilitated our year-round endeavours, always supporting rather than hampering our closeness to the earth's elements.

Our routines, uniquely tailored to our individual desires and capacities, reflect the very personal nature of this journey. Your nature's gym is singular to you, an adaptable protocol that honours both the season outside your window and the ebb and flow of your internal tide.

Motivation, that mercurial flame within, has been tended to with care. Through the undulating year, setting and tracking seasonal objectives has empowered us to transcend the sometimes-gloomy veil of seasonal affective barriers, emerging ever more vibrant on the other side.

Nutrition too has been foundational, a testimony to the ancient wisdom of eating with the seasons. Our bodies, much like nature, crave synchronicity with the cycles of the earth, drawing vitality from the harmony between what we consume and the climate in which we find ourselves.

For those who've ventured solo into the depths of nature's embrace, we've traversed the psychological landscape of solitude, finding strength and precaution in equal measure. Groups too have discovered solidarity in collective sweat and laughter, underscoring that human connection often deepens with shared exertion under the open sky.

Families have woven nature into the tapestry of their shared memories, recognizing that fitness and a love for the earth can be a legacy passed from one generation to the next. Cities, often seen as nature's antithesis, have proven to be ripe with opportunity for outdoor fitness, turning pockets of green into oases of activity.

In seeking the untamed wilderness, we've embraced the raw essence of the earth, shedding the trappings of our day-to-day to find clarity and peace in the wild unknown. Even beneath the canvas of the night sky, we've discovered a different sensory world waiting to be explored, revealing that darkness does not deter but rather enhances our experience.

And as we turn to mindfulness and wellness, nature has been the grandest of teachers, showing us that serenity often lies in a simple breath taken amidst the rustling leaves, in a moment of stillness balanced upon the earth's humbling foundation.

Yes, we are the thrill-seekers, the adventurers who edge ever towards the horizon, using the weather as a conduit for safely pushing personal limits and embracing a healthy form of risk-taking. Our path has undulated across mountains and valleys, yet we have also stepped lightly, ever mindful of the environmental impact of our pursuits.

Even when outdoor comradery wasn't possible, we've found sanctuary indoors, fostering an environment that resonates with the outside world. And as for the future, it gleams with possibilities as we balance emerging technologies and trends with a steadfast commitment to the purity of outdoor fitness.

Now, as we approach the trailhead of our own continuous excursions, the year-round call of the wild persists. It does not wane nor wither, but resonates stronger with each answered call. The wild, in all its seasonal finery, in its fiercest storms and its most enchanting tranquility, awaits. So let's step out once more, for the wild is not just a place, but a way of being that thrives within each of us, seducing us back, time and again, into its open embrace.

Appendix A:
Seasonal Checklists and Planning Tools

Much like the continued cycle of the seasons, our journey through embracing the outdoors for physical and mental vitality is never-ending. With each turn of the leaf, whether it's the fresh blooms of spring or the crisp air of winter, there's a cornucopia of opportunity to engage in activities that both challenge and invigorate us.

Springtime Readiness:

- **Equipment:** Inspect your gear from head to toe. Are your running shoes ready to hit the puddled pavements? Is the waterproofing on your jacket still resisting those April showers?

- **Activities:** Plan for the longer days. Maybe it's time to dust off that bike or start a running group that can relish the extra daylight.

- **Goals:** Set actionable and inspiring goals. What's been whispering to you over the winter months? A 5K, perhaps, or mastering a new outdoor skill?

Summer Structure:

- Hydrate, then hydrate some more. Prepare your water bottles and hydration packs for those sweltering workouts.

- Invest in sun protection. From tech-infused clothing to broad-spectrum sunscreen—prioritize your skin and eye health.

- Be water-wise. Have you considered trying a water sport? Kayaking or stand-up paddleboarding can be refreshing ways to train in the heat.

Autumn Adjustments:

- **Layer up:** As the temperature dips, layering your clothing allows for flexibility in your exercise routine. Think about base layers that wick away moisture and insulating layers that retain heat.

- **Low Light Prep:** Check your reflectives and lights, as the days shorten to ensure you're seen during your outdoor activities.

- **Trail Time:** Consider shifting some of your workouts off the road and onto the trails. Autumns canvas is perfect for a hike or cross-country run.

Winter Wisdom:

- Quality over quantity. With challenging weather conditions, it may be about shorter, more intense workouts to maximize exposure to daylight and minimize risks of cold-related issues.

- Balance indoor and outdoor activities. Have a plan for when the weather is too harsh—perhaps an indoor climbing wall or yoga session for these days.

- Self-care is crucial. Winter can be tough, but with a solid plan, including warm-up and cool-down routines, you'll maintain flexibility and prevent injuries.

Within these checklists, we find the skeleton for our year-round outdoor engagements. But don't forget the flesh and blood of this endeavor; your spirit, enthusiasm, and willingness to adapt. Keep your mind open to what each season has to offer, and equip yourself with the resolve to keep moving, regardless of weather's whims. Each season brings its own unique beauty and challenges, and with this guide, you're prepared to meet them head-on and embrace the ever-changing gym that nature provides us.

Don't let the thrill of the outdoors wane as the year cycles on; use these carefully curated tools to plan and keep your experiences both varied and full-hearted. Remember, with every sunrise, there's a fresh chance to align nature's rhythm with the beat of your own adventurous heart.

Appendix B:
Resources for Further Reading and Exploration

After diving headfirst into the transforming world of nature and the profound impact it can have on our overall well-being, it's natural to seek out more resources. Whether you're yearning for a deeper connection with the outdoors or you're simply hunting for that next riveting read, Appendix B is your treasure chest of go-to materials. It's time to expand your horizons and deepen your journey into the embrace of nature's gym.

Books are a superb place to start. They can be the gateways to understanding the subtleties of the seasons or the foundations for building your fitness amidst the elements. Look for books that interweave personal narratives with practical advice; tales of adventure with the science of well-being; and those that provide structured programs alongside open-ended inspiration. Works that touch on the psychology of solitude and the dynamics of group activities in an outdoor setting will further harmonise your understanding of the intrinsic human connection to our environment.

But don't just stop at books. The world is at your fingertips with the myriad of digital **blogs and online publications**. They're the pulse of the latest trends, gear reviews, and are often a vibrant community for sharing experiences and tips. Look for online resources that are updated regularly, honest, and, most importantly, that resonate with your own values and perspectives on outdoor fitness and exploration.

If a more structured learning approach tickles your fancy, there's a plethora of **online courses and webinars** out there, ranging from wilderness survival skills to guided meditation sessions in nature. These can offer a fantastic complement to your reading, providing you with direct guidance from experts you can interact with.

Films and Documentaries

The visceral power of visual storytelling can't be understated. A compelling **documentary** can teleport you to the farthest reaches of the earth or deepen your appreciation for the smallest patch of urban greenery. Watching others embrace the challenges and joys of the outdoors can spark that same fire within you to seek new adventures.

Podcasts

For those who are always on the move, **podcasts** can be your best companions on long walks or while conquering that steep incline. A good podcast can educate, entertain, and often feels like a casual conversation with an old friend. There are many dedicated to outdoor fitness, environmental consciousness, and the soothing sounds of nature itself.

Organisations and Clubs

Remember, learning doesn't have to be a solo activity. Look into joining **local clubs and organisations** that align with your interests. Whether it's hiking, bird-watching, or conservation efforts, being part of a community can greatly enrich your outdoor experience. These groups offer workshops, events, and the priceless value of shared knowledge and companionship.

Libraries and Bookstores too, remember them? Yes, the good old brick-and-mortar ones. These often host events with authors, have reading clubs, and the staff is usually more than eager to recommend a good read tailored to your newfound passion.

So, don't hesitate to venture beyond the last page of this book. There's a universe of resources just waiting for you to explore. Let this guide be the starting point, and let your curiosity lead the way. Whether through the written word, the shared experiences of a community, or the visual feast of a film, there's always more to learn and even more to enjoy.

Embrace this next stage of your journey with an open heart and a keen mind. The call of the wild is ever-present, softly echoing with the turn of each page, the click of each link, and through every interaction with fellow nature enthusiasts. So keep reading, watching, listening, and most of all, keep stepping outside. This is just the beginning.

Appendix C:
Safety Guidelines and First Aid Tips

Dive into the wild with confidence, knowing you're armed with essential safety guidelines and first aid tips. Let's not beat around the bush, communing with nature is invigorating but not without its risks, and a little know-how can make all the difference when you're out there pushing your limits.

Get to Know Your First Aid Kit

First and foremost, acquaint yourself with the contents of a well-stocked first aid kit. Whether it's a scrape from a rugged trail or a bee sting that threatens to sour your adventure, be prepared. Keep your kit accessible and ensure it includes antiseptic wipes, bandages, adhesive dressings, blister plasters, a roll of tape, scissors, tweezers, and pain relief meds.

Always Plan Ahead

Leaping into an impromptu jaunt may stir the soul, but prepping for potential dangers keeps you alive to tell the tale. Inform someone about where you're going and when you intend to return. A map, compass, or GPS can be your best friend in unfamiliar terrain, even if you're convinced you've got an inner homing pigeon.

Weather Wise

You wouldn't step into a blizzard in shorts or face the searing sun without a hat, right? The same goes for understanding weather patterns and preparing with the appropriate gear, as detailed in earlier chapters. Sudden changes can occur, especially in mountains, forests, and open water—so check the forecast and gear up accordingly.

Know Your Environment

Each season throws its unique curveballs, from hidden roots beneath fallen leaves in autumn, to slippery surfaces come winter. Education is your ally—learn what to look out for. Research local wildlife, too; from snakes in summer shrubs to ticks latching on during spring hikes, being alert and informed is key.

CPR: A Vital Skill

Cardiopulmonary resuscitation (CPR)—it's not just for lifeguards. A cornerstone of first aid, CPR can be a lifeline when someone's breathing or heartbeat stops. If you haven't learned already, consider attending a course. You never know when you might need it to save a life, possibly even your own.

When Blisters Strike

Blisters can take the spring out of your step. If a hot spot emerges, clean the area, apply a bandage or blister plaster, and if safe to do so, pop them with a sterilised needle to relieve discomfort. Never tear off the skin, it's nature's best bandage until healing progresses.

Bug Bites and Stings

Out there, you're fair game for mosquitoes, bees, and other bitey critters. If they do nip you, clean the area with soap and water or an antiseptic wipe, apply a soothing antihistamine cream or take a dose orally to quell the itch and swelling. Allergic reactions are rare but urgent—seek immediate help if breathing becomes difficult or swelling is severe.

Heat-Related Illnesses

When the mercury rises, so does the risk of heatstroke and dehydration, particularly during those scorching summer workouts. It's not all just perspiration and perseverance; sip water regularly, rest in the shade, and drape a wet cloth over your neck. Feeling dizzy, nauseous, or confused? It's time to retreat and rehydrate.

Cold Conditions

Remember discussing the beauty of winter's touch? It's enchanting but can bring forth frostbite and hypothermia. Layers are your best defence, but should the cold bite, warm those affected areas gradually. Shivering uncontrollably or starting to slur? You need to warm up, pronto, and seek help.

So there you have it—a snippet of the wisdom to equip you with confidence as you answer nature's timeless call. Embarking into the great outdoors is an unbeatably holistic experience for well-being, provided you step with care and respect. Whether you're facing the blaze of the sun or the crisp kiss of winter, remember: safety isn't just about survival, it's about making the most of every heartbeat thudding in tune with nature's boundless rhythms.

Appendix D:
Weather-Appropriate Recipes
for Outdoor Athletes

If you've been journeying with us through the chapters, you're well aware that each season poses unique challenges and offers rewards to outdoor athletes. Regardless of whether you're soaking up the sun or battling through a blustery blizzard, your body needs the right fuel to perform at its peak. This is where we've gathered some invigorating and nourishing staples tailored to support your body's needs in various weather conditions.

Summer Sizzle: Hydrating Smoothie Bowl

When the heat is on, you'll need something to cool you down and replenish lost fluids. This smoothie bowl is chock-full of antioxidants, natural sugars for quick energy, and fluids to help you hydrate post-workout.

- 1 frozen banana
- 1/2 cup mixed frozen berries
- 1 tbsp chia seeds
- 1/2 cup coconut water (or regular water)
- A handful of fresh spinach
- Toppings: sliced fruit, nuts, and a drizzle of honey

Blend the first five ingredients until smooth. Pour into a bowl and top with your favorite fruits, a handful of nuts for protein, and a drizzle of honey for a touch of sweetness.

Autumn Harvest: Hearty Lentil Stew

As the weather cools, your body craves warmth and substance. This lentil stew hits the spot with protein, complex carbs, and fibers that support sustained energy release - perfect for those longer, cooler outdoor activities.

- 1 cup dried green lentils

- 2 carrots, chopped

- 2 potatoes, cubed

- 1 onion, diced

- 3 cloves garlic, minced

- 1 litre vegetable stock

1 tsp each of cumin, coriander, and smoked paprika

Sauté the onion and garlic, add spices, and then the lentils and vegetables. Cover with vegetable stock and simmer until everything's tender. This stew can be carried in a flask and enjoyed warm mid-hike or post-run.

Winter Warm-Up: Energising Oatmeal

When it's frosty outside, start your day or refuel with a warming bowl of oatmeal. Oats are excellent for slow-release energy, and with added protein and good fats, you'll have all you need to brave the cold.

- 1/2 cup rolled oats

- 1 cup milk of choice or water

- 1 tbsp almond butter

- 1 tbsp pumpkin seeds

- 1 apple, grated

- Cinnamon, to taste

Cook the oats as you prefer, stir in the almond butter for added protein, top with pumpkin seeds for crunch, and grated apple for natural sweetness. Sprinkle cinnamon on top and you're good to go.

Spring Rejuvenation: Zesty Quinoa Salad

Spring calls for light, refreshing meals that prepare you for activity without weighing you down. This quinoa salad is bright and full of flavour, offering a wholesome combination of proteins, vitamins, and minerals.

- 1 cup cooked quinoa

- 1 diced bell pepper

- 1/2 cup chopped cucumber

- 1/4 cup diced red onion

- 1/4 cup crumbled feta cheese

- Handful of fresh parsley and mint, chopped

Dressing: Olive oil, lemon juice, salt, and pepper

Mix quinoa with fresh veggies and herbs, add feta for a salty tang and a boost of calcium, then dress with olive oil and lemon juice for a punchy finish.

These recipes are designed to be practical, easily adaptable to your tastes, and suitable for on-the-go nutrition. They don't just fuel your body; they're part of the joy and rhythm of embracing outdoor fitness year-round. Whether you're a seasoned athlete or embarking on a new fitness journey, let nature's bounty be the building blocks of your energy and recovery.